Prelude

You notice something. You can't quite put your finger on it but you definitely feel it in your gut. Sitting together at the kitchen table, you notice a slight movement of his head. The fingers tremble slightly.

Thoughts enter your head. ***Is he becoming sick? Should I make a doctor's appointment?*** It disappears from your view and in your mind. Life goes as planned. I help him pick out his clothes. He gets dressed and I make sure he has brushed his teeth. All is complete and I run him down to the Day Program.

This isn't any normal day program. This is a place for adults with disabilities to hang out. Al, my brother, has the chance to feel independence. He can hang out with his buddies. He meets new friends.

He learns to play pool and how to get along with others. With him basically being with me all the time I feel it is very good for him to have friends of his own. He learns that he can get free lunches if he earns them. He sweeps the floor after lunch or maybe he will set the table for the noon meal.

Al loves to hoard his money. His idea of money is to keep what he can and spend it on himself. Spending it on others is not in his plan. I have worked with him for years about gift giving and he did give in to my wishes but not with smiles.

Al experienced so much at his Day Program. He was able to go see a movie at the IMAX Theatre. He was able to go to Tampa and see ballgames. He went to zoos and the planetarium. There was usually a specific activity geared for learning and enjoyment each week. The city that we lived in was so big. There were many businesses that donated tickets. The main one was the Symphonies. Al was lucky to get to hear some great music during these years. Every afternoon when I picked him up, he chattered nonstop about what he did that day.

I would give anything to hear that chatter today.

To see the sparkle in his eyes.

To see the smiles spreading from cheek to cheek.

Al and I usually visited a flea market on Saturdays. He would beam from ear to ear if he found a coca cola item for sale. Al didn't care if he had several of the same things at home. His mental challenges only allowed him to understand that here was something for sale with the words coke on it.

I tried to teach him about running out of room and not buying the same thing over and over. We made some progress but even today, now that he has ventured into the classic car collections, he still has the same desires but we try to work through them.

We always made a point to go out to eat on Sundays. We usually went for supper for his convenience. Al is very structured in his routine. I could count on a bad day if I tried to change things around. He had to have a nap each day. Therefore, on Sundays it was routine to get up and go to church. Go home and get something light for lunch. He would watch his TV programs until 2:30 pm and then it was his naptime.

He would sleep until 5pm and then he was up and ready to go to supper. I was always amazed at how he had an internal alarm clock. He knew when it was time to rise in the mornings or from naps with his own built-in clock.

He loved to go to a restaurant called Dutch Heritage. You have to understand one thing about Al. I started caring for him when he was the age of 51 years old. Because he had disabilities and mental challenges, his whole life he wasn't along so many times when the family went out to eat.
It wasn't, I hope, that Mom and Dad didn't want him along. I believe that Al just liked time by himself. He had some ongoing

2

issues with his Dad and I think he enjoyed the freedom of making his own decisions when he was alone.

The Dutch Heritage was a huge buffet type restaurant. At first when we arrived there, I got up from my seat to start selecting my food and Al sat there. I asked, "What are you doing bud? Aren't you coming?"

He replied, "I don't know what to do. I am scared." He started to cry and then it dawned on me he had never been to a buffet before. I sat back down and taught him all about buffet style and after our first visit to the place I never had to teach him again when we returned.

He took so much pride in choosing his own foods. I sit here and smile as I think back to how he would fill his plate. It didn't matter how many times we visited, he ate in the same order. His food was arranged the same each time. He would get ham, macaroni and cheese, cole slaw and mashed potatoes and one big roll.

He only went up to fill his plate once. I think he always thought that if he went back twice he or I would have to pay a second time. After our meals were eaten, the waitress would always come around and ask what we wished to have for dessert. Once again, Al would look me in the eye with his starry eyes and with big pride beaming from his soul; he would make his own choice.

Always the same though out of all the choices. *Cherry pie with ice cream on top*. Oh, those Sunday memories I have with him. Seeing him, learning, and enjoying freedom of choice were some of the best times I ever had.

Chapter 1

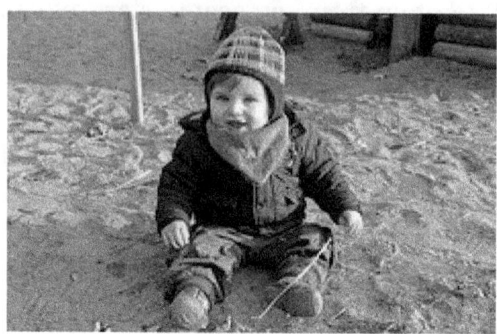

Al is my brother. I am one year and two weeks older than he is. My hope is that telling this story will help others who are struggling in their own lives to see that I am here and you are never alone.

It was May 3rd 1955 when a little baby boy was born. He did not come into the world welcomed as many children do. He came born into the world as an innocent babe by parents who had major issues of their own.

He was born with brain damage. He was the second of two children and this lead to lack of care needed to help a baby grow. As I remember back in my memories I don't remember him as much as I wish I would have...but the truth comes out over time and I will tell you what I was told.

When Al was old enough to sit in a high chair, he was placed there and ignored. No adult supervision. Al was able to maneuver himself up and over the high chair and fell different times causing more damage to the head.

Both Al and I were abused. In those days, it was not called abuse. It was a family secret that was only spoken of in strange moments. Al was abused more than I was. I think it was not necessarily that I was wanted more than he was. I believe it is because one baby is easier than two.

Our parents were not in control of their own lives. With their young ages, there was lack of training and maybe a feeling of entrapment over being strapped with two babies and a job that could not take care of all the needs within a family.

Parents of the parents stepped in and made opinions known. Guilt became an obsession and the need to escape became uppermost in the minds of our parents. Our Mother didn't work because she was too young. She was 15 when she had me and 16 when she had Al.

Dad worked at a bowling alley and hid behind the bottle when not at work. I have heard horror stories of how loud fights and beer bottles flew over our heads, as we seemed to be always in the middle of all arguments.

One day our Mom took off with us kids. She didn't tell a soul she was leaving. When Dad found out she was gone his Mother was grateful but insisted he get us kids back. I don't know with whom Mom left, I assume a friend took her. At her age, she wouldn't have had many adult friends to turn to. Back in those days, being pregnant and unmarried was taboo so I am sure the conversations were limited.

I know that while we were prisoners of my Mom's travels she had no money. She did whatever was necessary to survive. I don't know how she fed and clothed us kids but I do know that life could have been different when I was about two years old. I shudder to think what may have happened to Al also. There are parts of me that don't want to know. It is possible that Al can remember but it is so deeply hidden in his mind we may never know.

The Welfare department did eventually find us and return us to our Dad who was by now living back with his parents. Al and I were welcomed there simply because we were the "kids". I am not ever going to swear that we were united because of a great love.

I can remember sitting at my Grandmother's table and the room always being filled with silence. Grandma would tell him, "Be quiet. I can't stand that noise. I wish you would just shut up". I know that somewhere inside this house the word caring was lingering throughout. I know that my Grandparents took Al to the biggest children's hospital in our state to find out what was wrong with him.

I can remember them telling other family members that he couldn't sit up properly for his age. That he should be walking now but wasn't. The hospital confirmed that he was mentally challenged. He also suffered from Rickets and he was malnourished.

I don't think I was near as bad as he was medically. I do remember Grandma stuffing vitamins in eyedroppers filled with Iron to each of us kids. I am sure that we were both fed much better than we were before.

Al slept downstairs where my Grandparents slept. Our Dad still worked at the bowling alley and came home very late. I remember that I slept in a baby bed for probably too many years. I also remember that my Dad slept in the big bed next to my crib.

Eventually Dad met our new Stepmother. After being married, they moved to the town that Al and I now reside in. Visits came from our real Mom and I can still see me hiding behind the living room chair taking peeks at my real Mom and hearing them arguing about how she was going to come back to get me when I reached the age of 16. There was never a mention of coming back to get Al too. I can remember feeling confused and not understanding why she would only ask for me when I had a brother.

Dad then got a job at the State Highway Department and I think our new Mom worked at one of the local grocery stores. I remember she took us to a baby sitter. I knew fear even at the age of four. This babysitter was mean. I could see her smack Al for crying and I had to sit on a chair.

Yet there was a familiarity to this also. Al and I were not allowed to be kids when we lived at our Grandparents either. We had to sit on chairs and be very quiet. Neither of us knew what sunshine was or running and playing outdoors felt like.

Chapter 2

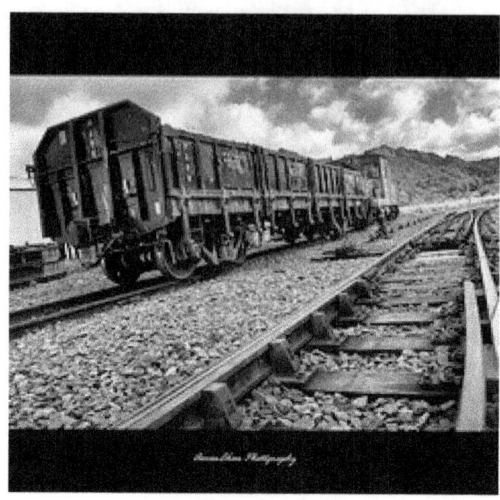

Al and I were introduced to our step-grandparents and these were very good times in our lives. Our Granddaddy as we called them lived in town in a big white cement brick house. It seemed like it took up the whole block.

It had a wraparound porch and I can remember sitting out there with Granddad many afternoons when he was home. He was a furnace man. He installed new furnaces for customers and many nights during the winter, he had to go out late at night to fix some person's heat.

Granddaddy had floppy ears and big brown droopy eyes. Al and I would crawl on his lap and he would always let us without hesitation. He talked to us and played with us. It brings me smiles now just thinking about him.

I remember seeing Al happy too. Grandma and Granddaddy took great care of us and spoiled us with lots of good food. I remember one time I waited on a white rickety square stool and watched my Grandma making a Black Raspberry pie. She took the left over crust and rolled cinnamon and sugar in it and baked them right along with the pie.

I couldn't wait to eat a slice of that pie. Even when it came out of the oven, I could barely sit still waiting for my own piece. I remember Al was four and I was five now. Waiting for a piece of pie with ice cream on top was pretty hard to do.

When I finally bit into the first piece, I can still remember starting to cry as I told Grandma that there were bones in it. You should have seen her. Her belly shook as she laughed so hard. She told me those were seeds and not bones. That pie still remains my favorite today.

We lived within the same block that they did. We lived in an even bigger house than Grandma and Granddaddy. I remember being scared every night when I went to bed. There were four bedrooms upstairs. I was the only one who slept up there. Al slept downstairs as he needed more watching over than I did, and yet I was the biggest baby of the two of us.

I lay up there many nights afraid of the trees casting shadows on the walls. I dreamed of people being in my room. I always seemed to be afraid of the night and darkness. The only thing that I really recall that was funny about that house is watching Dad use one of those old push style mowers. They were hard to work and he sweated a lot when he sat beside me on the porch steps to rest. One particular day when he and I were talking after he mowed a big old nasty bird pooped on my dad's bare back.

I know that I laughed and laughed so hard. Dad said some kind of cuss word that I didn't recognize but I didn't care. I was sitting with my Daddy, just him and me. I idolized my Daddy. He was God to me and never did anything wrong.

The other thing I recall is sitting in that small back bathroom that was behind the kitchen. Mom always thought sturdy. She had bought me black and white saddle shoes. I hated them with a passion. So when I was using the potty I would swing my feet back and forth. As soon as my shoes came into target range, I would spit on them. I told my step-mom about it when I grew up and she laughed with me.

Al always struggled walking. He had skinny little legs. He didn't run and play too much. He liked lying on the floor and lining up those little hot wheel cars. For a few years, Al wore Buster Brown shoes for toddlers. Mom always told me they helped his balance. I thought they were silly because he wasn't a baby anymore. He needed red Keds like the ones I had on.

I tried to teach Al how to use the hoola hoop but he never did get the hang of it. Al and I played a lot together. There was always some type of bond and I didn't have a name for but it was as if we understood each other.

I began to realize at a young age that I didn't need as much help as Al. I could do more on my own, so I became his big sister and pulled him in our big red wagon. I pedaled our big trike and Al stood on the back so he could ride too.

Al cried every time he had to have a haircut. In fact cried isn't an accurate word. Scream is more like it. I don't know today what the connection was but when he saw and heard the clippers he screamed bloody murder. I was always along and I bribed him with one-cent bubble gum pieces but Mom always said no. I guess he always swallowed the gum.

He also screamed bloody high pitches when we were sitting waiting at the train tracks for the train to pass by. I can remember Dad always yelling at him to "knock it off. It's only a train". I can still remember trying to figure out why Dad would yell at Al when he was scared. I would wrap my arm around Al and tell him, "it will be alright baby brother. It *is* almost gone". Al sucked on one of those pacifiers and he used to offer me a suck from it when I made him feel better. Somehow, even back in those days Al knew I was there for him.

Chapter 3

Al and I were lucky for a few years while our Grandparents lived in the big white house. We had cousins who lived very near. Parents would take us trick or treating. Al would never wear a mask. He would scream bloody murder. I never knew what he remembered in his mind but something had made him deathly afraid of so many things.

Mom would dress him up with old clothes from home and would leave his head and face untouched and we would go out and trick or treat. Al didn't want to go up to the doors so I would always get a couple of extra pieces and put some in his sack too.

I can remember Al and I used to sit for what seemed hours staring at the silver tinsel Christmas tree. It had one of those moving lights under it and the tree changed colors. All the ornaments would sparkle and I can see Al still smiling so much with those big blue eyes.

When school started, we went to the same school. However, by the end of Kindergarten Mom and Dad knew that the school we attended could not help Al. He was switched in first grade to a school about three blocks from my school. I walked to school and a special bus came and picked up Al.

He went to the Special Education classes all through elementary grades. These years seem blank to me. He and I were separated for the first time. Different teachers and different programs. I do remember Al going with Mom and Dad to my school activities and me doing the same at Al's school.

One thing that comes back in my memory is the big fan. In Grandma's house, my Granddaddy hung a big motor fan over the screen door. I used to love to sleep on the couch in the summers and I was lulled to sleep by the noise of the fan. I still use a fan today and so does Al.

One night although it was a school night Al and I got to stay all night at our Grandparents. We were awoken early in the morning while it was still dark. Granddaddy told me that we had a new baby sister.

I don't remember being thrilled over this. By now, I was ten years old and it had always been Al and me. Now we had a sister. I knew that everyone was excited but Al and me. Of course, he didn't understand what that meant that we had another sister. He already had one, me. I felt a little bad inside because I wasn't sharing in the excitement.

Changes happened then with our family. We moved away from the happy block. We moved a few miles away. I wasn't able to see my Grandparents near as much, which made me sad. Al played more and more on the floor being very quiet and lining up all his hot wheel cars.

I turned to my baby dolls and pretended I was the mommy. I didn't realize it then but somehow now reading back what I am writing I see that something bad had happened and I needed to be told I love you. I in turn told my baby dolls I loved them. I fed them and changed their diapers and clothes. I pushed them in the baby stroller. I couldn't fit Al in the baby stroller so I pulled him in the wagon and continued letting him to ride on the back of the big red trike.

An old woman started watching our new baby sister, and eventually we slipped into that group. Al became more into himself and I started to change too. I would cause problems. I would eat so much junk and then blame it on others. I went so far that I raced in from the garage when we got home and I would open drawers and flip over chairs and then when Mom saw it, I stood back and snickered as she questioned the neighborhood Moms about where had their kids been while we were gone.

I must have been really messed up over the baby sister. It seemed that this is when I began to look at Al as my brother and Dad as my hero and the baby sister as the unwanted.

Al and I were never really involved with the new sister. Al started doing worse at school and he started stuttering. Mom used to have to go into the school that he went to for meetings. She always yelled at Al on how she worked full-time and he needed to straighten up so she didn't have to be away from home so much.

I doubt that Al and I knew what really was happening back then, but I do know that Al and I stuck together more and more. It was us against the others. Al didn't only start his stuttering. He had started getting something called impetigo. It would start on his lip and sometimes it would grow all over his chin.

I can remember Mom picking at the scabs and me yelling at her in my 10-year-old voice to quit hurting him. He was crying and I would run into the bathroom to see why he was crying. She made him cry. She was always picking at his face. I am sure she thought she was helping to get those ugly scabs off. *But what about his tears? Didn't it matter that he was crying? Please leave him alone Mom. Don't make him cry.*

Chapter 4

I remember Christmas the following year. Al got a train set. It had a soft whistle. I think Mom and Dad were hoping to calm his fear of trains. The track went around the Christmas tree and I can still see Al lying on the floor watching the train go round and round. When Dad made the whistle blow Al did not cry.

Mom and Dad were very smart in this idea. It worked and in time, Al became less and less afraid of trains. Our entire extended family spent Christmas together. I still have photos of my two cousins in their new striped bib overhauls. The silver tinsel tree is standing in the background.

The next year Dad received an inheritance from a family member who passed away. He and Mom decided it was time to move our family out to the country. I didn't realize exactly what that entailed. I was excited because I was going to get my own bedroom.

Al and I had slept for a year or two in the same bedroom in bunk beds. Now a hallway would separate him and me. When the house was finished, it seemed that Al and I parted a little bit.

He stayed in his room a lot and I rode my bike in the summer and went sledding in the winter. Al did eventually learn to ride a bicycle. He was so proud and he would ride up and down the country road. He would have freedom to choose to stop in at Grandma's house or ride back home.

I should add that our Grandparents sold their city home, bought 80 acres, and a home. It was shortly after our parents built a house a quarter of a mile down the road. Another neighbor that happened to live in the same city block that we all did also bought a house on the same road.

I always laugh when I think back to how four neighbors living in the same block and not all related ended up buying or building all within walking distance and remained for years to come.

Al was now 11 and I was 12. This year started the big change for my brother. Our Granddaddy was in seventh heaven having the dream of farming come true. I can remember watching baby calves and pigs being born.

Granddaddy had the patience of a saint. He took Al with him everywhere he went on the farm. He taught him about life. He was silent while Al worked at becoming more vocal. Dad was already showing that he was uncomfortable around Al. I always believed that Dad carried guilt from our birth years and shame that his one son was not like other sons.

Carrying these feelings caused great stress in our family. Then Granddaddy would come along, swoop Al up, and take him to a calmer environment. While he taught Al and me how to pick up baby chicks, he also taught us how the circle of life works with farm animals.

We bottle fed new calves, we gave water to baby chicks. Al even laughed aloud as the baby lamb drank milk from the bottle Al was holding. We were shown how chickens laid eggs and then how chickens ended up on our kitchen tables. We were taught that calves were grown to feed us and to purchase more farm animals.

Granddaddy taught us that living off the land was the only way to go. I will always treasure these times and Al still talks about Grandma's big, soft, chewy sugar cookies. They were as round as grapefruit. If we were very good, we could have two at one time. Sometimes Al got three but I understood what Grandma was saying. Al was skinny and needed to eat.

She made the best ever potato salad too. Lots of big pieces of boiled eggs in it. She used mayonnaise in hers and Mom used a vinegar sauce in hers. I preferred the sweeter one and still love my sweets today.

I remember one time when Granddaddy was cleaning out the barn where the cows lived. He was cleaning the manure with his pitchfork. Al wanted to try it and so Granddaddy handed him the

15

pitchfork. Al wasn't too strong at this point yet and he got a fork full and then fell right in it. He started to cry and Granddaddy laughed him right out of his tears. All three of us got a good laugh over this and Grandma was stuck cleaning Al up.

These farm loving Grandparents were not our blood relation, but I can tell you that they were the best ever, and when you talk about them to Al today, his eyes always light up, and for his memories that he still has of them I will be forever grateful.

Since three families lived on one big property there was a great big garden. All summer long canning and freezing was done. Al got the jobs of taking garbage cans of corncobs to the pigs. He had sort of the gopher job, but yet it was one of the most important jobs. While everyone had their hands in food, Al would go get things that everyone needed.

Sometimes when we worked very hard, our Grandparents would take us to the Dairy Queen. We would get great big ice-cream cones. I will share with you something that will tell you a difference between our parents and our Grandparents.

Grandma worked at home, taking care of family and gardens. Our mom worked full-time. Granddaddy was laid back and enjoyed every minute of breathing. Dad was always afraid Al and I would make mistakes so he was always on edge. When Dad was dating our new, mom-to-be it was in the fall and early winter. Dad would bring us two kids along but made us stay in the car. He truly did believe that we would make noise. Grandma would yell at him every single time and tell him to "go get those kids out of that cold car".

When our Grandparents took us to the Dairy Queen, we all went in and we made messes because by then Al and I were both big gabby mouths. They would laugh at us and talk with us. When we were finished, we all cleaned up and went home laughing.

When Mom and Dad took us to the Flagpole to get ice-cream Mom was antsy because Dad was always on the edge of yelling. She became embarrassed for Al and me as Dad made us stand outside and eat our ice cream. He didn't want any accidents.

I always felt bad for Mom. Although it took me many years to bond with her, she was an excellent Mom and she cared about us kids. She did the best she could with what she had considering Dad was always a grouch, but she loved him for a long time.

Chapter 5

We lived up on a hill with lots of trees surrounding the house. It was a great hill to go sledding as long as you didn't run into those trees. A couple of times I took Al down on the back of my sled but he never did like it and seemed scared. He preferred to be in his room playing with his cars. Al played with his hot wheel cars far later than most kids, but he loved them and he was never asked to put them away and grow up, which I am thankful for.

In the summertime, Dad always made him trim the trees. Oh, Al really hated this. I am not sure if he actually hated the trimming or if he hated the fact, it was Dad telling him to do it. We were never allowed to ask questions. If we didn't understand, we could go to Mom if she was there or we just figured things out for ourselves.

For Al no matter what the project was he needed training longer than most of us. He would in the beginning trim around the trees but not close enough. So Dad would go out there and show him again by pointing to the trees and asking, "Do you see now what I am talking about? Now go back and redo them all".

Al would cry and Dad would walk back to the house shaking his head. Dad shaking his head was a common thing I saw clear up until his death. He never understood why we kids just didn't get it the first time.

This is when Al learned to start cussing. I sometimes would go out and walk with him while he did the trimming for the second time and I learned some choice words. I will never know where he learned them at that age because neither of us were allowed to hang around anyone that didn't go to church.

I can remember when I wanted a friend to stay the night. Mom would ask, "What's their last name"? If she recognized it as a bad family name, I wasn't allowed to be near them let alone have them spend the night at our house.

I guess when I look at it Mom she was prejudice. You were hung before judged if you had the wrong last name. I can remember the house that was occupied by people other than Caucasian. Mom would always say, "Don't step in the grass or ever go in the house on your way home from school. They have bugs".

I laugh at it now because it sounds so silly to me. *How did her mind work?* I always blame it on her upbringing and what she was taught. I didn't get mad at her, I always listened to what she said, but I made my own judgments when I became an adult. Any human can get bugs and your last name means nothing to me. I will decide after I have taken the time to be with you whether we would make good friends or not.

By now, Al had outgrown the special education classes and was in the high school. He really struggled. Fears that had been held at bay now resurfaced as he struggled with stuttering and learning disabilities.

I am not sure what Mom did but I know she spent a large amount of time in our school. A class opened up for students that were labeled back then as slow learners. Before that, it was called mental retardation.

I always hated that wording. Even today, when Al is down on himself he will sometimes call himself a retard. I jump on him quicker than you can blink an eye. I tell him in no way is he retarded. I explain that some things are just a little harder for him to learn.

He and I are both left-handed people. I always tell him how smart he and I are. That we are the lucky ones because God only gave left-handed to special people. Then he would smile at me and the world was good once again.

The new school class was an ordinary class but a few special need students were placed in here. Not only was there a teacher but there were two teacher's helpers too. I always told Mom she started a revolution for learning disabilities with whatever she had said to get this started.

Mom was never one to brag about herself. She worked as a manager for a big well-known heating company. She paid people's bills when she learned that the customer was trying so hard but couldn't pay the entire bill. She never let anyone know it her that paid the bill.

Mom even helped to open the first women's shelter here in our town. It was for women and children who had been battered by their husbands. It is still running at high capacity today unfortunately. I say this because I wish abuse of any kind would fall off the earth and never be heard of again. We learned, we conquered, and now we lay it to rest.

Al stayed in this class the entire year and we could start to see changes in his personality. He was feeling like he was cared about and that teachers understood him. He stayed in these high-school special classes until he graduated. We were all so proud of Al for graduating. He should have graduated in 1973 but instead he graduated in 1975, but hey, who cares, he made it!

Chapter 6

This week could have been better for me. I have suffered minor setbacks of almost panic attack feelings. Stress and tight muscles as I went to bed and waking in the mornings to the same feelings. I wondered if I even slept well at all through the nights.

This has been happening to me ever since the day I thought Jesus was standing very near to me. I think that my mind races like a spinning top about all kinds of things. Al coming home soon. *Will I be able to do everything I need to when he is here? The inner guilt of choosing Al over working outside the home. Wondering now that I have written a few chapters what really happened to Al when he was little?*

It just seems I do not stop the thought process, and I have learned to hide beneath my covers and sleep. This doesn't help me long-term. I realize it is a temporary fix but at times, it is enough to relax me some.

As I was about at my wit's end last evening where I just wanted to pull my hair out, fall to my knees in tears, then a good friend of mine from Canada called to chat. She told me that she felt she was supposed to call.

God has the perfect timing. He knew that I had enough. My bucket was ready to spill over and he sent a friend to the rescue. We talked for over an hour. I almost didn't want to talk at first. It is very difficult for me to release the silly feelings that I carry inside. It is much easier for me to pretend that life is good and all is well.

My friend is a very strong Christian woman and so I was able to confide in her questions that had been spinning in my mind and we talked through them. By the time we hung up my tight chest had relaxed and I felt an inner peace I had not felt all of this week.

She made me see the light about caring for Al versus having money in my hands. She told me that God would take care of my needs as long as I am sincere. I feel very sincere when I say aloud; " I want my brother home with me. I want to give him all the support I can. I want him to know that he is loved and I will be here with him through this journey of his life".

Maybe once Al is home I can get the routine down pretty well and pick up a job caring for someone else while he is at Day Program. I dare to say that my first book is now done and getting ready to be published very soon. *Would this book make me any money? I didn't write it for that reason, to get rich. I know that is a foolish dream*.

I wrote it for my children for when I am no longer here. I wanted to leave a mark here on earth, a memory of how I think, but if God wanted me to make money off it, I will. He is an amazing God and whatever he wishes for me will all be good.

I think one of my deepest thoughts that fly around in my head is Al. When I read back what I have written, I see what I was put through at a very early age. I see how my innocence was stolen from me. But, what about Al? Surely, there are reasons that he was so afraid in those **young years. I don't believe that children are born afraid. Something or someone has placed that fear.**

My friend and I prayed together over the phone that God shows me how to help Al release the hidden fears he has kept buried all of these years. I can do nothing to help him alone. I have tried so many therapy sessions with him and we get nowhere. However, God can do anything.

It won't help Al rid the disease of Parkinson's disease. It could release bad memories and bring him a release and therefore joy. Seeing Al carry joy in his heart and the two of us leaning on each other cannot do anything but help us both.

Knowing that Al believes in his heart that I really do love him would be wonderful. To see him trust me totally would be so wonderful. So now, I ask the Almighty God to help me to help Al.

Chapter 7

After Al graduated, I was out of the picture off and on. I had been married and lived in Germany for a year. I was expecting my first child. So thoughts drifted in and out of my family life and my new family to be.

When I came home to the States Al had a number of jobs. This is when a new set of problems started. Al had money of his own. A real paycheck that he wished to spend however he wanted.

However, life doesn't work this way. We have bills and most of us cannot take our money and spend it entirely in one week. Al didn't understand this. His thoughts were, he made the money, and therefore he could spend it as he wished.

He had a car payment and auto insurance. I admit life was much easier when Mom was around. She felt bad for Al because he didn't make too much money for his hard labor. She often helped him and swore him to secrecy.

Even with Al's mental issues, he understood that this secret was to his benefit so he was always quiet about it. Al went to several jobs for quite a few years. He worked in a factory but he was fired. He was too friendly with the ladies and he would smile big at them. Often he would tell them they were pretty. These women did not like this and thought he was weird so they reported him and he would be fired.

This went on at a few jobs like this. He worked in egg manufacturing where he had the dirtiest job of all. He had to clean up at the end of the day the mess of cracked and spilled eggs from the machines and the floors.

I always felt bad for him. He worked very hard but because he was mentally challenged, his pay was much less, right at the minimum wage. *I thought it was unfair but the companies always said the same thing.* "We can't get the same production out of him as we can the others".

Some of the other jobs he had he just plain talked too much. He has always been a social butterfly and will speak to anyone who looks his way. He is still like this today if he is having a good day.

I think Mom got tired of all the jobs so she talked to our Aunt and Uncle. They owned a meat market. Meat was brought in, butchered, and packaged up. *Once again, in my opinion, Al got the crap job.*

I won't say it killed him but gosh darn, it was a hard job they gave him. He was responsible for taking those half beefs off the racks in the coolers and bringing them out for butchering. *Do you have any idea how much one of those weigh? My Dad told me once that a cow weighed 1000 pounds. That is a lot of weight for one person. Many times, I watched him do this.*

For high season work when deer were bring processed I would work there helping to wrap the finished product. My job was much easier than Al's and I made more money than he did. I could go on and on about how it isn't fair to under pay a mentally challenged or disabled adult, but I won't. It would take me another chapter.

One day the small family business closed and Al was out of a job. Mom got Al involved with a company that helped to hire and house disabled adults. The first thing the company did, and I will call them C.C. for short was to do a month-long load of paperwork.

After this was completed, they moved him into an apartment living situation. It was run through C.C. and Al was given the title of Client from then on out. He lived in his hometown with three other gentlemen.

They found him a job a half an hour away. It was a veal farm. I am not sure what he actually did, but I imagine anything that he was asked to in the barns. He got very homesick.

He was too far away from home. He missed his own bedroom but Mom urged him to keep trying it. She was sure he would adjust and learn to love the freedom he was allowed. Al never learned to cook. He is deathly afraid of fire and so never wanted to learn to use the stove.

I believe the way it was set up is that each of the four people had special knowledge of one thing or another. When you put this all together, you had a house that was clean and the clients were fed.

One time Mom paid a visit to Al and she went into shock when one of the guys let her in. There was Al and a female client from another C.C. apartment sitting on the couch together. They were holding hands and watching a pornographic movie on the VCR machine.

Mom didn't believe in this at all. Even at home, when I lived there I saw Mom one time in her slip. Walking around half-dressed was neither allowed nor proper in our home. Cussing was not allowed either. Mom was a God-fearing woman and very strict in this area with us kids. I remember one time Mom was so mad at Dad that she said shit.

I thought I would die laughing when I heard her. What a naughty word that was. Mom's excuse was, "He just makes me so darn mad. I shouldn't have said it and make sure you don't say it either".

At this age, I had definitely already said it before but I wasn't going to tell her. Well, she told Al to get up and get in the car. She took what she could take on that trip and took him home. She went back and got the rest of his things and then when she got home she made the phone call.

"I saw my son in a position that may lead to sexual encounters and he was watching that sex stuff on his VCR. I'm sorry, he can't live there anymore. You don't watch him good enough. I have him home now. I will call tomorrow and make an appointment to see what other options we have".

Chapter 8

Al never did move away from the family home again. I think Mom had just had enough. Him being so homesick and then the nasty movie he was watching. I felt Mom believed he was better off at home with her watching over him and keeping him in a good church.

By now, I was back from Germany and my husband and I and our daughter had rented a small home about a mile or two from my parents. It was out in the country and I loved it, but I loved more that I was close to Mom and Dad.

Life went about the same for several more years. People got sick and healed. There were birthday celebrations and the holidays. Mom used to make Al and me an angel food cake. She would use this frosting recipe called

Seven Minute Frosting.

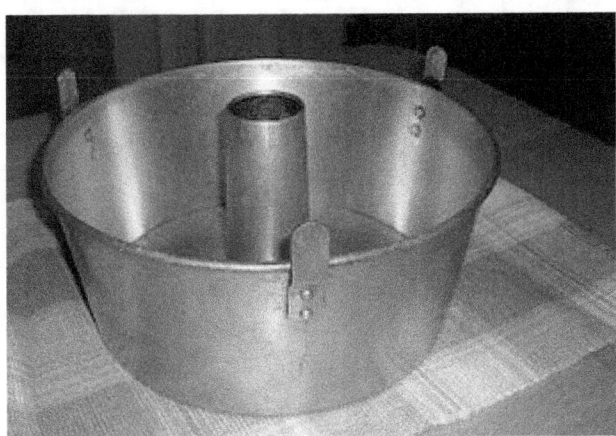

Original recipe makes 2 layers (filling and frosting)

- 2 egg whites
- 1 1/2 cups white sugar
- 1/3 cup cold water
- 1 1/2 teaspoons light corn syrup

- 1 teaspoon vanilla extract

Directions

Put egg whites, sugar, water, and syrup in top of double boiler. Beat until
mixed well. Place over rapidly boiling water. Beat constantly with electric beater while it cooks for 7 minutes or until it will stand in peaks when beater is raised. Remove from heat. Add vanilla. Beat. Fills and frosts 2 layer cake, 8, or 9 inch.

We kids loved this frosting. The first day you ate it, it was so light and fluffy. Mom would tint it blue for Al and pink for me. With the size of an angel food slice and all that heaping frosting it was a kid's delight. She also added those candy decorations on top. Remember those? They came on a piece of white paper that you wet the back and then the candies came off. They had letters, flowers, and candleholders. When you are a kid, biting down on those crunchy candies was so much fun.

Christmas was so much fun. Al got trains for Christmas to help him get over his fear. I got baby dolls. I remember getting a Baby Thumbelina one year and another year I received Chatty Cathy.

Mom and Dad loved buying us gifts at Christmas. Dad got the biggest kick out of watching us open our gifts. He loved to Christmas shop. Our special gifts were always unwrapped under the tree and I can still see Al and me racing to the tree to pick up Santa's big gift.

One year Al and I opened a homemade marble game. Al was fascinated by it much more than me. He would spend hours and hours dropping the marbles down the maze of zigzag shaped slots. All the marbles would eventually end up in the bottom in a flat tray. Then he would do it over and over.

We always spent the holiday with all of our family. Then through the year as the family got smaller, we started going to Mom and

Dad's on Christmas Eve. By now, I had my own family and we always enjoyed her homemade lasagna and homemade candies.

Then when it was all over my family would go home and put our kids to bed. After they were asleep, we would finish doing their gifts for the next morning.

Al lived at home so he, Mom, and Dad would have their own little Christmas in the early morning. Al never knew what to buy anyone. He would go to our Grandma's, our mom's mother and she would write down ideas for him. He still struggled, so one gift per person was written, and then he would go buy it. Grandma would always wrap his gifts for him and he would tuck them under the tree.

Life changed for Al quite a bit when Granddad passed away. There was no one but Grandma who went out of their way to help Al with all the problems he had. Mom worked and so did Dad. Granddad had Al with him all the time, and then suddenly he was gone.

Our whole family changed. Al was more alone and there was so much sadness floating throughout the house. Now when Al went to Grandma to talk or get help with a problem for a few years she just was lost without her spouse and we became lost in her world too. Not by choice but she was mourning.

Dad had to start doing more for Grandma plus his own job and I think he became tired. He started jumping on Al's case easier and it became more often than before. Mom spent her free time with her mom who was still mourning. I didn't live there any longer, and our

Half-sister never got along with Al.

I know for me that I was so jealous of our sister. Even though I understand much better now that I am older, I didn't get it then. She got new clothes from more expensive stores. In fact, she got almost everything she wanted. She went with friends a lot. She seemed to have quite a few over niter parties. While Al and I were much more quiet. However, we have to remember that Al and I were ten years older than our new sister was. We had been taught to be quiet, while the sister was laughing and much louder.

I think Al never knew what to think of her. As he saw himself being yelled at for being stupid, he never saw her in trouble. I think in Al's mind this bothered him and he felt less wanted than he should have. He always felt like he was the bad kid and he was in the way.

Chapter 9

Al started spending more and more time at Grandmas. She lived on the same property as Mom and Dad did. In fact, the property was large enough that it held three houses and each house had a family member in it.

When Granddad passed away, Al was asked to go down and spend the nights with Grandma for a while to help ease her pain. He had no trouble with this request. He loved Grandma very much.

It didn't take long before a routine developed. He would go to work each day and then he would go home, shower, and then head to her house and the two would eat supper together.

Suppers at our own house were never pleasant that I can remember. I can understand why Al went the other direction. At our house, I could never put my finger on the problem. I know it really wasn't us kids directly, but maybe it was and we didn't realize it.

There was always tension, so thick you could cut it with a knife. If I wasn't being forked in the elbow for bad manners, Dad was picking on Al for anything that came to his mind. I never remember Dad ever saying, *good job Al, I know you did your best.*

What I remember is, **why can't you ever do anything right? I tell you and tell you over and over. Do you have something wrong with your brain? Are you just plain stupid? I may as well have done it myself.**

Through the years that I lived there when I was still growing up or even when I would drop over for a visit and end up eating a meal with them, this never changed. I used to say to myself, **Well why don't you just do it yourself then and leave him alone.**

Mom would get all tense and nervous through these meals. Mom had a great outlook on life but Dad always ended up tearing it down.

I don't know if Dad meant to or even knew the stress he was causing.

I knew they had arguments behind bedroom doors. I hate to think that Dad was intentionally being mean. I think he felt so insecure about his own self he couldn't stop it. Back then, you didn't run to the therapist for every problem. You fixed it or lived with it.

Mom worked the 8-5 job and although I cooked many meals and tried my hardest to keep the house cleaned, it was never enough once we all sat down at the dining table. Our half-sister was the adorable one. She talked about school and what activities she was in. Conversations quickly turned to her to escape even more fog.

When I graduated from high school, Mom and I weren't the closest. I always knew that she and I had never bonded like moms and daughters should. I loved her best I knew how, but she hurt me.

I pondered on what it would be like to have a Mom who really loved me and wanted me. I am not ever going to say that I didn't cause grief for her. I think most kids cause grief for their parents.

I moved out of the house and got to be one of those bratty kids according to my Mom because I didn't remain at home. My Mom worked up town and I would sit across from her office on the courthouse lawn and watch her through the window.

Why did I do that, I don't know for sure. I think now when I look back I wanted her to notice me. I wanted to make her feel as uncomfortable as she had made me feel. One summer day I was sitting on my favorite bench and I walked over to say hello to her when she got off work.

I walked with her to the back alley where her car was parked. I don't remember what transpired between her and me but I do remember those cutting words even today. "I don't know why you can't be like your half-sister. She never gives me trouble like you do. But of course I could never love you as much as I do her. She is my only child".

Wow, what a blow to me that was. I think deep inside my gut I knew that was the way she felt about me but to hear the words. I wanted to run and hide under a big rock. I wanted to die right there on the spot.

I tried for years to forgive myself for ruining her life. It never worked. Then I blamed her thinking, *well no one forced you to marry into a ready-made family. Don't blame me for this.*

I wonder now as I write this if Al understood enough and felt the way I did. We were the extras. We were the baggage that came along. If she wanted to marry our Dad, she had to take us in too.

Mom told me one time a few years before she died, "you understand Terry, why I could never adopt you and Al and legally be your Mom. I was always afraid of your real Mother coming back for you if she read or heard about it".

I can remember looking at my brother Al, and in my heart telling him, *it's not our fault bud. We didn't ask for this. You and me, we belong together, we are real brother and sister. I love you bud.*

Life for me became more dismal after she said that remark. It sliced so hard and deep that I still haven't gotten over it today. While I am writing this, the pain instantly re-surfaces and I feel the deep ache of wanting to belong.

I have to believe that inside Al's head today is masses of memories too difficult to deal with. They remain hidden and buried so deep that even with all of the professional counselors I have had him to, nothing works.

Counselors do alright until they touch the subject of parents and Al flips out. I don't mean slightly, I refer to him as a tornado. Dark and huge coming at you with daggers so sharp they would kill you.

The topic was always dropped when the professionals saw this. They usually dismissed him as a client also. We went through five therapists. The last one specialized in Adult Disabilities and she just knew she could help Al. Once again, when she approached the parent topic after having seen Al for one month, he exploded.

I never tried again after he was so outraged that the police were called and they had to calm him down by force. When I hear the word therapist today, I use every block I have within me to keep Al safe.

I know that he should get it out of his head, but I refuse to put him through hell ever again. God will deal with Al. God will protect him in the perfect way. I do not have what it takes to approach this subject matter. When the nursing home came to me with the idea of someone speaking to Al, I stood tall like a fence and said, "NO!"

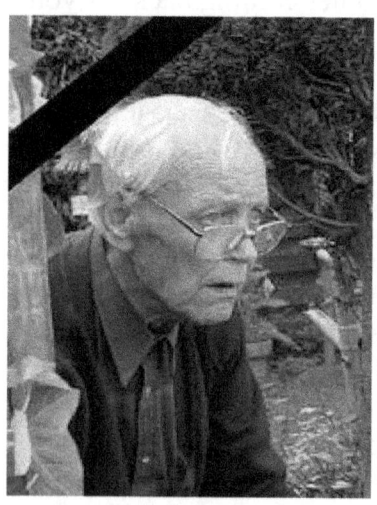

Chapter 10

Seeing Al today at the facility brought old memories for him and none for me. When I walked down the long haul, I could see him immediately at the dining table. He looked exactly like I never wished him to look. A stare across his face, head bent down and frozen somewhere in time.

When I approached his table, he barely looked up at me. Once I got our food settled that is when he began to cry. I asked his nurse how he had been all morning, and of course I already knew she would say, *fine, just fine, no problems*.

I wanted to run away but I cemented myself to the chair. I was feeling like I am the one who makes him cry. I am family and this brings back memories for him. He was back in time. While I was living a married life, I do remember Al getting the opportunity to go down to Indianapolis, Indiana to the big Memorial Day races.

He has told me several times in the past about the fun he had going to these. When our Uncle Jim was still alive, he had as much patience with Al as our Granddad did. There was always a bond between these two men and Al.

I believe in my heart that these two men saw clearly that our own Father was not being the best he could with Al. They took many times and fit Al into their fun schedules.

Today, Al cried the two hours I was there. He spoke of the race, but he could remember very little of it. What I remember from earlier years of him telling me about it; is that they chattered all the way down to Indy, a three-hour trip. They left at 4:30am, and Al always says, he didn't have a problem getting up that early, it was worth it.

They filled up on hot dogs and sodas. They saw wrecks. Al told me of the speeds of the cars and who was driving what cars. Today all he could remember is that he went with Uncle Jim. It broke my heart, it really did.

There was a time when Uncle Jim and his wife moved to Florida. They went there because one of their children had Cystic Fibrosis. The air was to be better for him. Although Al had never gone anywhere alone, after graduation of high school, Uncle Jim arranged through the airlines for Al to come down for a visit.

All arrangements had been made with the stewards and gate crew to keep a good eye out on Al without Al realizing it. He made the trip with flying colors. He always said he had a good time.

For years life seemed to be monotone for our family. I was raising mine and Al remained at home. He helped in the gardens in the summer, shoveled snow in the winters. He worked from job to job and then finally landed a job where he worked for nine years before he had his heart attack.

Al and Dad kept their distance or when they were together, it was pure hell. Dad would yell, scream, and threaten. Al's face would turn beet red and his fist doubled up, his body tense and ready to attack.

Nothing ever changed. Different family members and friends tried so many times to help Dad see the damage he was doing to Al but Dad brushed them all off. I am going to add my own personal opinion at this point.

Our non-blood Grandma and Granddad and our Uncle Jim and his wife, were not directly related to us, but they were the best back in those days. They all spent great deal of quality time with Al. Helping to nurture him and grow into a man. I used to hear from my Dad's sister how she used to have to help take care of us when we were brought home from the kidnapping days.

I will call her T. T said that she used to give me a bath quite often. I don't know how old she was, but evidently a teen. She told me of the day she scalded me and how bad she felt about it. I am sure it did bother her and I hope she moved past that. I never remember words of anyone speaking about the care Al got. The only times I can recall any talk about Al is when he had to be taken to the Children's Hospital for rickets and undernourished.

When I became a teen, I was alert enough to realize that there is a word called fake. You have family members that can say all sorts of nice things, but when you aren't in the room, you can eavesdrop in on the truth.

Cousins used to laugh at Al. He was mildly mentally handicapped. He wanted to fit in. He wanted to laugh with others, speak, and carry on with everyone. Usually, the only one laughing out of innocence was Al. The others were laughing at him. It always hurt my feelings because I believed that we were all family, and this was a bad behavior. I noticed that Al was left out of many things.

When there were reunions or family dinners, Al was placed at the kids table. When everyone was playing Badminton, or croquet, Al was not asked. Card games, he was in the room watching television. I always wondered if he realized he was being left out.

I sure wish I could put a photo up of my brother from early days, but I have never seen even one tiny photo of him. The ones I post on here for you to see look to me like he is maybe five. *I wonder why no photos were taken or if there were, where are they?*

Before our real grandmother passed she handed out all her photos. Anything that had to do with our family I got the pictures, but none of Al. I have my baby picture but I gave it to my daughter. Maybe we didn't really exist in people's minds until my Dad and Stepmom got married. Maybe we were the kids, who were in the way, the two that were from a broken home, or maybe the two who were kidnapped. Something happened. Photos show pride and there are no photos of Al or I except the one baby picture of me until after my new Mom came into our lives.

Chapter 11

For most of Al's life after the teen years, everything remained the same at home. Mom and Dad worked full-time. Al went from job to job. He would lose a job because of not comprehending quickly enough what needed to be done.

He was let go from a couple of places because he spoke too much to the ladies. From what I was told, the ladies were scared of him. Evidently, they were not used to being smiled at and having someone say hi to them so often. In the past, I have heard people; strangers make remarks about "The Freak". Oh, that made my blood boil

I think we all have issues in life. It is just for some, it is obvious by looking at them, and others, it is not so noticeable, like repeating the word hi to the same person every time they walked by. He still does this today. He just wants so badly for someone to be friends with him.

Cardinal Center is a company that helps disabled adults get jobs, and this was an excellent program for Al. He worked at the same job for a long time. During this period of his life our Step-mom and it is going to be here that I quit calling her this. I will call her mom. I have spoken about the real mom but she doesn't exist in our lives. In fact, Al never even remembers her.

So it was at this time that Mom was retiring from her job. She stayed home for some time but eventually missed being busy so she went to work for a health company taking care of their payroll. After a few years went by, she finally retired for good. The next week she had an aneurism.

Dad found her on the potty and called the EMS. Our Mom never drank, cussed or smoke. She was only 62 years old when this happened. She was taken to the local hospital where she stayed for several hours and was then transferred to a bigger hospital about an hour away.

While she was at the local hospital, Al and I were there with her. Al didn't really understand what was happening but he knew something was wrong. I will never forget Mom thrashing her arms and legs around on the ER bed. She managed to get her arm out to me and she kept patting my arm. It was almost as if she was telling me to be strong; it is going to be alright.

That was the last time Al and I saw her conscience. By the time they got her to the bigger hospital, she was unconscious. She never came out of it. I lived at the hospital per say, and Al came up before he went to work. Seven days later, the doctors told Dad and Al, our half-sister, and me that Mom only had 10% brain activity left. "Did we want to keep her on a breathing tube"?

Our tiny family huddled together. Al and the sister didn't say anything. Dad and I decided to let her go. After they unhooked her, Dad was watching me the entire time while he and I held her hand. It was as if he was asking me, is she ok?

It was a sad time for us those next several hours. Finally, I was the one chosen to go tell Al that she went to heaven. Al didn't cry. Instead, he went into himself even further. The rock that held our family together was gone.

From that, moment on Al had no one to speak to. Shortly after Mom's funeral was over, my aunt in Florida moved her mother down to that area. Dad became withdrawn, and Al was left to figure out how to survive.

He went to work and came home alone. He ate alone and watched TV alone. He and Dad didn't even sit in the living room together to watch TV. When I tried to reach out to Al, Dad would tell me to butt out.

Dad believed that if everything was going fine then don't mess it up. However, things weren't going fine. Al was suffering and so was Dad. Al started going to auctions out-of-town and this is when he really began to collect his coca cola.

Dad hated it that Al was spending money. I will never know why. Dad charged Al a small amount of rent money for living there. I never agreed with it but I couldn't stop it either. Al barely made above minimum wage and he already had a car payment and auto insurance to pay for. Dad even made him purchase his own groceries.

It was so stupid. Dad put his refrigerator items on two shelves and Al put his items on the other two shelves. They were not allowed to mix. *It makes my skin quiver just thinking how sick that was between a father and a son.*

When Dad and Al went to church it was the same one for a while and they each drove themselves. Then Al changed churches. Nothing they did was together. Dad got so upset with Al spending his Saturday evenings going to the auctions that he finally had his friends go to the auctions too and spy on him.

I thought so little of these people that they would disrespect Al so bad and even stoop low enough to do as Dad wished. I hated knowing this was going on but again, I could do nothing.

There was no one to stand up for Al anymore. *What his life must have been like for him I can only imagine in my own mind.* I felt so bad for him but I was forced to live my own life.

After several years of this routine, Dad finally met a new lady friend. He introduced her to Al and me. She seemed very nice and she was pretty. Dad liked it that I agreed with his selection. Al didn't say too much but the little he did tell me was, *that's not my mom.*

Chapter 12

The new lady in our Dad's life seemed so pretty and nice. But she was a snake with a poison tongue disguised in fine linens. Dad was guilty of sharing with her issues he had most of his life as they became closer.

The one thing he did share with her, and for name's sake, let's call her B. Dad told her many of his frustrations with Al. He never took the blame for his feelings. It was easier to place it on others.

Dad would tell her how Al fought to trim the yard, but he omitted to explain Al's mentality and slowness. He told her that Al would not mow the yard, but again he never said Al had never mowed because he was incapable.

It wasn't long before B decided Al was a piece of crap, disappointing his Dad, defying what his Dad needed from him. She took it upon herself to lecture Al any chance she could get. The catch was she always did it behind Dad's back.

She could smile oh so pretty, but away from Dad, she was a venomous snake ready to pounce. I have to be honest here; I think even if she had said something in front of Dad, he wouldn't have done a thing.

Dad was always afraid of what others thought of him. He was always ashamed of us kids. It is so hard to explain to you because even today I don't myself understand why. *I know he loved us, well, I am pretty sure he did.*

Al learned to hate this woman B. He would run and hide if he found out Dad and B were coming over. I say coming over because by now she had invited him into her home to live. This left Al was once again on his own. Dad and B would come over to mow or check the mail. While Dad mowed, B would go into the house.

I can still remember once when I was there to see Dad I walked in on B yelling at Al. She was saying," You are such a disappointment to your father. Why do you fight him so bad? Don't you think you are old enough to be out there mowing instead of making your sick Dad do it? No wonder he moved in with me. He needed to get away."

I stepped up to the plate and threw her ass out. I told her, "Don't you ever talk to my brother that way again, or I swear you will regret it the rest of your life. Now get the hell out of our house."

She and I never told Dad of this conversation. You see Dad was sick. He had Bone Cancer. I didn't want him to have the added stress in his life. Another thing I should add here is there was five acres to mow with a riding lawn mower. Al could never have done it, even if he had tried his best. With his coordination, he just wasn't capable of doing this chore.

B treated me different at first; nice is the word I would say. She was the pretty one. She lived on a beautiful piece of property on a channel. She had a cute little dog and kept an immaculate house. She was not going to be taking care of a sick man. She would cook for him but that was it, and he could sleep in her bed. Other than that, it was all up to me.

I took Dad to all of his doctor appointments. I took care of insurance companies. I had a job where I went to work at 6pm on Friday nights. I lived at this house taking care of an elderly married couple. I would leave Monday morning at 8am and return that same day at 6pm. I stayed all night then left Tuesday morning at 8am. Then I was off the rest of the week.

In between this job, I took care of Dad. I would be invited to Thanksgiving but Al wasn't. This was just eating me alive. I was actually invited to the dinner because I was his caregiver and she was his lover, cook, and housekeeper. I had to be there in case he needed something.

I was there quite a bit. I took care of Dad from March 2007 until he passed away in December of the same year. B would take him on

42

leisure one-day trips and of course, I had to go along. Al would go to our Aunt's home for holidays and I would be with Dad and B.

I guess at one time B and our step-sister had met and got along fine and once again Dad had confided in his disappointment in her and B sent her away too. Therefore, I was the only one allowed in her home and even then, I knew the only reason was that she needed me.

As Dad became more ill, I was there more and more. I was asked by Dad to come over more often than not. I think from his and my conversations he knew that he had made an error with picking her but was too afraid at this point. He didn't want to go back to his home and die alone.

Dad was a big part of the blame for B not getting along with Al and the other sister, because he never cleared up the truth. He let her go on and believe what she wanted. As I was at her home almost constantly to care for Dad, she would say hateful things to me.

I felt so torn. Dad didn't want to go home and live. I had begged him to go back to his own house and I would care for him there. I told him I would get coverage for part of my hours but he insisted I stick with my job since I was almost divorced from the now ex.

Chapter 13

Things at B's house became more fragile, the longer Dad was sick. The more time that went by the more, he wanted me to be his caregiver exclusively. I would be at work and I would receive calls night and day.

Thankfully, I worked for a wonderful family. I had actually known the kids way back when I was a teen. I had run around with one of the daughters. Even if the call came through the night, I would call my boss and let her know. She would say, "Go ahead Terry, run over to him, and then come back as soon as possible." I was running three different lives as caregiver all at once, but I did it. Anytime Dad called, I was there.

By this time, the half-sister and Al were completely out of the picture. Al has a routine he follows. It is part of his mentality. As long as he doesn't have to part from this, he is alright. He went to work. He worked at a linen company and worked from 10am to sometimes 7 or 8pm. It was sort of crappy hours but he didn't say much. He would come home and eat one of his frozen chicken patties and I don't know what else. He watched TV and then went to bed at 11pm each and every night.

I would call and check on him but was still not allowed to actually go in the family house. It was one of those situations. I was forced to look at as a fight or flight. I thought, *as long as I know he is alright, I will let things rest, while I take care of my husband and wife team and Dad.*

When I would go into B's house either to play cards with Dad or be his caregiver, she or the dog always met me at the back door. As soon as I stepped into the kitchen, she would start in on me.

"I am just so damn pissed that I am with a dying man. Do you know what we did when my own husband was dying? We all got a beer and gave him a beer and we would sing around his bed and get drunk."

I just looked at her in awe. I couldn't imagine this but of course, I was not and still am not a drinker. I have seen the damage alcohol can do to people. Don't get me wrong, I am not here to criticize, but in my opinion, I want to know the stupid mistakes I make in life.

I never said anything about her remark and let her proceed to belittle me all for the sake of Dad. She would show me the cupboard full of medications and express how Dad was taking up her kitchen space.

She would show me the partial bottles that I needed to call the doctor on or go have refilled. She would show me her refrigerator and tell me how many dollars she spent on Dad just trying to keep in here what he wanted to eat.

She said she was on a limited income and could not afford to give him whatever without the fear of going broke. From then on, I would call Dad on my way over and ask what he was in the mood for to eat, and then I would go get it.

As he became weaker, he always wanted egg-drop soup from the Chinese Restaurant. That became about the only thing he would eat, but it was alright. He would have me feed it to him and we chatted and gave each other eyes for words.

B got bolder as time passed by. She would begin to tell me about their sex life. *I hate to tell you this, but I wasn't interested in Dad and her sex life. For heaven's sakes, this is my father we are talking about.*

After while I wasn't even sure if she was telling the truth, as Dad couldn't make it up her staircase anymore, and if she did get him there, she pushed him all the way up the stairs. I was just standing by, holding my breath, waiting for him to fall backwards and topple on her and they both would come crashing down, but it never happened.

Then she began to tell me what a disappointment I was to my Dad. I heard things I had never even questioned in my own heart that I had done to hurt him. I knew that I had disappointed him in some ways.

45

We always want more for our kids than we had and maybe I didn't produce all he wanted, but I loved him and accepted him for all his faults. He was my hero; I had always placed him high on a pedestal. I don't feel this way any longer after caring for Al.

She would tell me bad things about Al and the sister. She would complain about my Mom. *This used to make me royally pissed. She never even knew our Mom. Mom had died seven years prior. I wanted to tell her off so bad but alas, I couldn't. I wanted her to be out of the picture. How I thought she was so nice and pretty in the beginning is beyond my own imagination, for I now looked at her as the wicked witch of the west.*

One time when I was at work she called me around 1am and told me, "Your Dad is wet. If you want him dry, you had better get your ass over here. I am not changing some sick man."

I would get up out of bed and make sure my people I was in charge of were alright and then sneak off to the five-mile trip to her house to change him. I would not see her when I arrived. She would leave the back porch light on and the door unlocked. I used to think, *why hasn't someone broke in here and kidnapped the old hag?*

After cleaning him up I would race back over to the house, I resided in on the weekends. After work ended, I would run by Dad's house and make sure Al's car was gone. Relieved, I would head home to try to live some sort of life.

Chapter 14

As Dad got worse, Al became farther back in the picture. I liked it better when he was fore most in my mind because he needed looking after. However, B. felt that Dad was just a big burden and demanded more and more of my time.

One of the last visits Dad paid to his own home, it was in October. He had the urge to sit on his tractor one more time. B. came along and I met Dad out at the house, Al was home also.

Dad made me go get Al, as he wanted to talk to him. It ended up not being talking, it was screeching about how things were not done the way Dad wanted them done. Our half-sister happened to stop by and my Grandma still lived on the property.

We were all getting things arranged in Grandma's house as she was planning to move permanently to Florida to live with her daughter. It was still pretty warm outside and the woods were in full color.

I didn't know how we were going to get the tractor out of the barn. Dad had tried to climb on top of it but he was too weak. Just then my son pulled in the drive way and I asked him to bring the tractor out.

While my son was, doing this B. was in the background bitching at Al because of this or that. I told her, "Stop it right now. You have no right to be speaking to him this way. Leave him alone and remember this is neither your son nor your home."

She gave me a dirty look and then proceeded to start in on our half-sister. It escalated very quickly and soon there was an arguing match in full force. I am so thankful my parents lived in the country. If we were in town, the cops would definitely have been called.

Yelling and accusing was going on so long. When I glanced at Dad to see how he was dealing with this he was sitting in a summer chair and his body was trembling. He was so weak and too afraid to interfere with this fighting.

I probably didn't handle it the right way, but I told Al to go ahead and go back in the house where he would be safe. Al didn't hesitate he left right away. I walked up between the sister and B. and stuck my hands out in between them. I probably looked like a traffic cop. I told them," You are destroying Dad. Look at him trembling. You two should be ashamed of yourselves. If you want to argue and bitch, go somewhere else and do it in private. I want this shit stopped now. I will not sit here and watch you all destroy yourselves."

Voices hushed and the air became quiet. B. was beginning to mumble under her breath and I gave her the look. She changed her train of thought, went to Dad, and told him she couldn't help herself. She just wanted to protect him. ***In my opinion, she could just shove it and go to hell.***

After the boxing ring became quiet, Dad went back to the issue of wanting to get on the tractor. My son and I tried and tried to hoist him up but to no avail. Finally, I saw a five-gallon container. I went and grabbed it and placed it as a stepping stone for him.

He was able to get on and he sat there smiling. He tried to start the tractor but his legs were too weak to clamp down on any pedals. Getting him off was even harder. My son and I balanced him and sort of pulled him off.

There was no more arguing that day. B. had said what she wanted. Our half-sister was done defending herself and inside Grandma's house. My son left, so all that was left outside was B., me and Dad.

I grabbed Dad's mail and we all went back to the girlfriend's home where I helped Dad inside. The day before when I had visited Dad, I had brought over a toilet commode. He could barely get down on the seat to sit or stand to be wiped.

I had the ability to grab him this and a walker. When we got inside her house and I had Dad seated and comfortable in his recliner, she called me into her kitchen. When I went to see what she wanted, she had the commode in her hands. She made me watch as she tossed it out the back door. She commented or hissed, "No one is going to pretend they are sick in my house. There will be nothing here that represents sick."

I watched her with intent as she tossed that and the walker outside. I went outdoors, grabbed the walker, and brought it back inside. With Dad within hearing distance, I played out a short clip of a silent movie.

I raised the walker and pretended I was going to slam her with it. She covered her head with her hands and inside *I was having the time of my life.* On the outside, I was firm-faced and I mouthed to her, "He needs this, admit, and now get your shit together".

She left the walker alone but put it on the back porch. I had to look at B. for the first time with sadness. Although I never met her husband who had passed, I could imagine the memories of having another man you cared about dying in your home once again. That feeling of sadness didn't really stay that long, as I knew that someone in her sixties should very well know better to take it out on another human being, no matter how bad it hurts emotionally.

Chapter 15

The more ill Dad became the more I was at the home of the girlfriend. I tried my best to be smiling and talk about nothing but it was strained. Dad was fearful that he or I would say something wrong and he would be sent home packing.

Many times, I heard B threaten to send him home if he didn't behave. I felt so sad for Dad. I always knew that he was not one of those take-charge men. Mom did everything. She paid the bills. She made the better money. She was very involved with the city of our hometown.

Dad stayed in the background. He had plenty of friends himself. The guys he worked with, and there were some from his church that he hung around with. But Mom always seemed to outshine on most things.

I always believed Dad had issues with Mom making more money and I feel that this hindered him taking a front seat in their marriage. So seeing this woman bully Dad when he was dying broke my heart.

Many times, I ate over at B's house. She was an excellent cook. Her home was spotless. Her dog was cute, the property she lived on beautiful. Nevertheless, she lacked in humanity. Her life revolved around her and we were the tagged children, and Dad was her puppet.

The minister started dropping over at B's house to see Dad more often. Dad made it a habit to read his Bible after breakfast each day. When the minister would stop by B made a fool out of herself my making rude comments to the Reverend. She would say, "He reads his Bible but he doesn't follow a damn thing in it".

I used to want to just walk over and slap her silly when she talked like that. I am sure both Dad and the minister were embarrassed. I know I was. After the visit was over, she would pounce like a cat all over Dad. "How can you be such a hypocrite? Reading that damn book and then not living like it says. You ought to just put it away somewhere and forget trying to look like something you aren't"

I don't care if she was right or wrong. She should have never voiced her thoughts to him. I have known our Dad much longer than she has. I remembered a time when he would not step foot inside a church door. He had changed. He needed and wanted to read his daily devotions. He counted on it. Dad did not want to die. He wanted to live. He did everything in his power to keep living. I think he clung very tightly to what he read each day.

Moreover, she and I nor any of us have any right to judge another human's thoughts. Who are we to throw stones when we have not looked in our own glass mirrors first?

I stayed with Dad pretty much through the weekdays. I went over in the mornings and stayed until after the supper dishes were done, then I would go home. On the weekends, I had to trust that B would behave as I worked all weekend long.

Spring, summer had passed and now it was fall. Dad wanted to go to a flea market. B drove and I tagged along in case Dad needed attention. When we arrived in the parking lot and we were ready to take off B let us know that she was going on ahead. She didn't have time to wait for Dad who was slow and using a walker.

Dad and I went into one tent and looked around and then he could go no farther. He and I sat in the shade of a hot fall day and talked while we waited for B to have her fun. On the drive home, I was very quiet. B talked and Dad listened.

That was the last time I went anywhere with Dad other than his doctor appointments. I am glad I had that time with him. While we waited on the bench, our talks began to become on a more personal level. Dad and I both knew he was not going to make it.

Thanksgiving came and it was a nice fall day. Of course, I was supposed to be there that day. Who else would give Dad his shots and medications? Who would help him to use the bathroom facilities?

I had a terrible time because I knew that my brother and half-sister were not with us. Thanksgiving Day to me means a day of being thankful. A day of being with family. My siblings were not allowed over. ***Oh how I hated her for this.***

I got a hold of Al and made sure he was not going to be alone on this holiday. I discovered he had been invited by Dad's sister to be at their home for dinner. For this, I was very grateful. I explained to Al how I so wanted him to be with me, but because of B's attitude it just wasn't going to happen. I apologized to him repeatedly and I don't think he understood or does to this day why he was left out.

The dinner table was filled and over-flowing with a turkey and all the trimmings. At this point in Dad's life, food was the last thing he wanted. He would rather be sitting in the pillow-based recliner that we had designed for his body.

When you are dying from Bone Cancer, even a button on a recliner touching your skin can cause great pain. There were many times that I could no longer give Dad a hug. The cancer was eating holes in his bones making him in great pain and very delicate. However, this didn't matter; he had to be at the head of the table. He was to pretend that life was great and the food divine.

If I remember right, he ate a small helping of Turkey and a teaspoon of mashed potatoes. Dad ignoring the homemade chocolate pie told any of us that knew him well that he was very sick.

He didn't want to stay at the table. He begged me to take him to the recliner. Although B was bitching about him leaving, I took him to his chair. On the way from point A to point B, Dad quietly asked me, "did you make sure Al is alright today?"

I said," yes he is. He is at your sisters."

It made me feel good that Dad inquired about Al. Things were changing inside Dad. He was beginning to take stock of what he had done in his life. What kind of father he been to Al. I think it was eating him up about certain things that had been left undone or unsaid. He touched my hand and said, "Thanks Terry for making sure he is alright."

Chapter 16

From the point of Thanksgiving until December 1st, life spun in circles. I didn't see Al for this period of time. In fact, I didn't see anyone. I worked my job and when I wasn't there, I was with Dad.

Dad and I had quite a few talks about things kids don't usually discuss with their parents, but Dad knew he was dying. He talked to me about Al and he discussed his personal will with me.

We didn't do anything when I was with him. I talked and he was quiet. I gave medications and the only time he would eat is when I brought him egg drop soup. His sister dropped by more often. She and B would spend time chatting and I stayed by my Dad's side.

On December 1st, Dad was in so much pain. He couldn't sit still. I was constantly changing him from the chair to the bed. There wasn't a position that was remotely comfortable for him.

He finally lay down on the bed. I didn't even think for one second if it looked bad or not. I lay down on the bed beside him and placed his hand in mine. He quieted down and for about fifteen minutes, we lay there with me telling him how much I loved him.

His eyes were closed but I knew he could hear my words. Then he opened his eyes and they became wide and then they closed and he took his last breath. Oh Lord, I will never forget that moment and five years later, I still re-live that moment over and over.

I got off the bed and went to tell his sister and B that he had passed. They had not been in the room with Dad and me. They were in the bedroom across the hall chatting. When I told them, they both said, "Really?"

They got up, went to where he was, and told him they loved him. I never felt as alone as I did at that moment. It was up to me to call the funeral home. I made that dreaded call, went outside, and sat in the swing and smoked. Crows filled the trees. Their chatter was so loud and when I looked up at the trees, they were black in color from so many birds.

As quickly as they had come, they left. The funeral home came and I could not go inside. I stayed out until Dad was removed from the home. I was so thankful to the parlor as they helped me decide things. Who was there to call was one thing.

Dad's sister's husband, my uncle volunteered to tell Al and our half-sister. While the attendant and me were making decisions I don't know what happened to B and the sister, but suddenly they appeared with Dad's wallet and they had emptied it.

I was in too much pain to notice or think twice about what they had been up to. I didn't even mind that Uncle was going to tell my siblings. The dust settles though and you learn of what was happening around you once your mind becomes clear.

Considering Al is disabled with mental challenges I would have made the effort to go to him in person and tell him the sad news about Dad, but instead the Uncle called Al. *This had to be the coldest move ever. I can only imagine how Al felt getting a phone call stating, your Dad is dead.*

Through the years of caring for Al, he has told me how awful he felt. He didn't know what to do. My heart still aches at the crappy way in which he was dealt the news. Just as bad as that the month prior to Dad's death Al and our half-sister were not allowed in B's house. Neither of my siblings were given the chance to say goodbye or settle any last thoughts with him.

I try very hard not to dwell on this topic today as the pain is instantly resurfaced and I find myself becoming depressed for a few days. That afternoon of his death, I went to the funeral home and tried to make plans with the attendant. My Uncle kept trying to take over and make the decisions. Finally, the owner of the home asked my Uncle to please, remain quiet. It was time for the eldest child to take care of matters.

I can remember the looks on their faces as this task was taken out of their hands. They were not very happy. I did my job. I let the owner walk me through the steps. I went to my daughter's home for a few days.

I wish today that I had handled things differently. All I can think of was my brain was fogged. I was moving out of habit but not thinking. Poor Al and the sister didn't have me around or my support. I am so ashamed of not being there for them. I was being led around hand over hand and questioned nothing.

The funeral came and the burial was over. I was made Executor over the estate and had plenty of work to do with this. I checked in on Al daily. I saw our half-sister much more often.

One week after we had buried Dad, I received a phone call from Al's family doctor. He was letting me know that Al had left his job and driven himself to the doctor. Al was having a heart attack.

Up to that point, my mind was on the continuing path of how life was before Dad's death. I was going to get Al an apartment where disabled adults lived. He would continue with his job and routine that he was used to.

This caused a knife into a bubble effect. Our lives changed at that moment and never went back. We were creating a new path in life, with gravel instead of paved. Big potholes and rather large bumps.

Chapter 17

My mind wasn't catching up to what was really happening. I had been visiting Al and trying to concentrate on my job. I couldn't get a handle on the fact that our Dad had died the week before.

Now I had this estate to take care of and the phone call from the doctor put my mind at a slow halt. What was I doing? What was I going to do? I immediately went to the hospital. I just couldn't believe Al drove himself to the doctor when he was having a heart attack.

However, I have to keep in mind that he was mentally challenged. All he knew was that he was hurting. Once I got to the hospital, it was confirmed that they were transporting him to Fort Wayne hospital where there was a heart floor.

I waited with Al until the ambulance came and then I stopped at the gas station so I could buy more smokes. I was a nervous wreck. I thought my head was going to explode. It was just too much at the wrong time.

I sped all the way. I beat the ambulance by a few minutes. Once I registered him, they prepped him for emergency surgery. It was after he was announced alright that being his sister was not good enough.

Here was a mentally challenged adult who had always lived with our parents. I was not his legal guardian so I fought for everything I wanted Al to have. After a few days, he was dismissed and I was allowed to take him home.

I ended up spending that night but still I was thinking *I will just keep a good eye on him. I will check on him every day. I can do this.* As I spent more time at the house, I discovered Al had such a good routine going that he didn't have any decent food in the house.

In the freezer were seven boxes of generic breaded chicken patties. You know the ones that you aren't sure if there is really any chicken in them. He also had several packages of hot dogs. *It is no wonder he had a heart attack.*

As I went through his room thinking I was just going to tidy up, I began to notice things weren't right. There were health issues here. Ever since Mom had died, Dad never opened the house again. Central air or heat was on all year round. The windows had not been opened in seven years.

I found white mold growing inside dressers, under the sink, on several floor moldings. I am a clean person and seeing this scared me for Al's health. I went home, got some clean clothes, and decided to spend a few days since I only worked Friday through Monday mornings.

Everything Al did was on routine. If his routine was messed up or changed Al was lost. He is mentally challenged in the cognitive area. This is the only way he made it for seven years after Mom died and Dad moved on with his life leaving Al to fend for himself. Al stayed with his routine.

He bought groceries on the same day each week. He ate the same food for breakfast 52 weeks out of the year. He packed the same lunches. He drove the same route no matter what the weather was. He went to ball games in the winter. He went to auctions on Saturday nights even if there was six inches of snow on the ground.

On the day that it would have been laundry day, I decided to help him out since he was healing from his surgery and so I gathered up his laundry and started to sort. I noticed there were no white clothes to wash.

I went back in his room and asked him where his undies were. He said," I don't have any. They all got holes in them."

" Well why didn't you go buy some more?"

" I didn't know I was supposed to," he told me.

***It was at that moment that some of my fog cleared and I realized Al
had been just getting by.*** I sat down on his bed and talked to him
about me moving in. I wasn't sure how he was going to take it. He
had grown so accustomed to hiding when Dad was home; I wasn't
sure how he would react to a new change and it being a family
member.

The conversation was fairly simple. " What do you think about me
moving in and helping you out while you get better? I could help
you pack your lunches and fix your suppers through the week."

That part must have interested him. Before our Grandma moved to
Florida to live with her daughter, Al always went to her home for
supper. He told me I could move in. I made sure he was going to be
alright for a while and then I went to my apartment and packed a
week's worth of clothing.

Without me realizing I was already beginning to take care of my
brother. For a few days, I spent my time between taking care of him
and cleaning the house. I scrubbed down mold, cleaned bathrooms,
swept, and opened the windows to get fresh air in.

Al had a doctor's appointment. I went with him so I could hear what
the doctor had to say. The doctor reported that Al could go back to
work on light duty. This made Al angry. He was concerned about
what his boss would say. All I remember Al asking was," What is
Scott going to say when I don't do my job? He will fire me, I just
know he will."

It took a while to get him calmed down so I explained to him that we
would go talk to his boss. I had Al go with me inside to where he
worked. I explained what was going on and they were happy to let
Al go back to work, even on light duty. Al felt better and the tears
disappeared. To celebrate I took Al to Wendy's to eat.

He had no idea what he was supposed to do. He didn't know how to
order food. He told me he didn't remember ever being on the inside

of a restaurant. I am sure he had been but it bothered me that maybe it had been so long he didn't remember.

Slowly I taught Al about the other part of life. The fun parts, other than work and sleep. I taught him how to understand the menu boards. I showed him how combinations came with a sandwich, fries, and a drink. It wasn't long at all when I would take him to eat he would stand right up there at the counter and say, " I want a 2." The employee and I would chuckle together because she was thinking that he was so hungry he couldn't order properly, but I knew that this is the part he understood and this was the way he was going to get food.

Chapter 18

Life seemed to settle down into a routine. Al worked Monday through Friday. I had breakfast for him, packed his lunch and had supper prepared when he came home. On the weekends, he had to take care of himself. I made sure there were easy foods for him to microwave and eat while I went to my job taking care of another couple.

It wasn't easy but I was able to juggle the Estate of our father, taking care of Al and doing my own work. Days turned into weeks and then the bomb fell for Al. I received a phone call from his job.

The conversation was pretty one-sided. I was informed to come in the next morning; we all needed to talk. Al was aware that something was going on. I think he had been having some issues at work. Since he ran on routine, he knew he was at work, but I knew he was aware he was not the same after his heart attack.

The next morning Al went to work as usual. I sat looking out the windows watching deer run through the field as I drank my coffee and pondered on what the meeting was about. *I had my suspicions.* I could see that Al just wasn't back to his normal self after his heart attack.

I finished my coffee and went and got myself presentable and then left for town. I turned on the oldies station, trying to deter my mind from bad thoughts about what was about to be said.

Reaching the parking lot and walking through the front doors I was greeted by Al's boss and other people who knew Al in production. I was guided into a meeting room where Al was already seated. Coffee was offered and I politely turned it down. I wanted to get this out in the open.

The office people smiled at me and then the conversation began. " We all love Al. He is just a real joy to have here. He will do anything that is required with a smile, but we have noticed that since these few weeks have gone by, Al cannot get his speed back up."

Others chimed in with affirmation that yes, they had also noticed. Then Al's closest boss started tearing up and stated," No matter how we feel about Al, we still have rules and regulations to follow here. We have given Al every opportunity, and through no fault of his own, his health will just not let him do his job properly. We must let him go."

Al understood this and instead of getting mad like I thought he would, he broke down and cried. Others followed his lead and soon everyone was crying and telling Al how much they loved him and would miss him. Each of them had some type of memory gift from the factory and then Al and I were led to the front door.

We walked to the car in silence. Once driving back home Al made one comment. " I am just plain dumb. I am retarded, just like dad said I was." I wept and tried it reassure him that he was nothing of the kind. I told him "We will make it through this bud; we will make it through this".

Al loved milkshakes so I offered to stop by his favorite place, Dairy Queen and get one. He turned that down and instead ordered a Blizzard. A mixture of Reese's Pieces and Reese's Peanut Butter Cup.

It sounded really good to me, so I got a small one, and of course, he got a large. He never went back to shakes again. It was a blizzard and the same type from that day on. We went down to the park at the lake and sat on the picnic benches with our treats. Neither of us talked. We just watched the ducks and looked out over the water.

Throwing our cups away, we drove home. Al went to his room. I tried to talk him into coming out in the living room and watching TV, but he had been trained to go to his room and so he wouldn't budge.

As I tinkered around the kitchen, I thought about choices I may have. *There didn't seem to be any choices. I knew in my heart that the right thing to do was to move in with Al full-time. Any ideas I had previously of moving Al into his own apartment where disabled adults lived I tossed out the window.*

Al didn't give me any argument. In fact, he went with me to my apartment and helped carry things out to my car. It was a small apartment. I had moved there after leaving my husband. I called it my Box Apartment, because it was so tiny.

It didn't take Al and I very long to get everything finished and by dusk, I was moved in. *I have to admit I felt a little uncomfortable. This was our parent's home. I had grown and left the nest. Now I was going to be sleeping in my parents' bedroom.*

After making sure Al was settled for the evening, I went to my parent's room and unpacked my clothing and bathroom supplies. I squeezed in my knickknacks between mom and dad's things. I did my best not to upset Al's routine. I left him alone to watch his TV and do his own thing.

I didn't need to upset Al though. He was confused. He thought he was a failure. He had been fired as he stated. No, he had no money, he thought. How was he going to go to his auctions? How was he going to have gas money?

Chapter 19

Al seemed bored through the days. I could understand. His routine had been broken so what was left. I did not work through the week so I started asking him if he wanted to go out to eat for lunch or supper. He never turned that invite down.

It took Al no time at all to walk up to the front counter and place his order. He was proud. Sometimes he would pay and others I paid. He would get the biggest grin on his face while he pulled out his wallet and paid for his own meal. He would sit the wallet on the counter and pull out the exact number of bills. He carried a sandwich baggie in his pocket and he would take that out and get the exact change. Al always had to be exact with whatever he did.

When we were home, Al stayed in his bedroom. Every day I would encourage him to come out and watch TV with me or spend time out of his room but he refused. His room was his refuge, his hide-a-way. He went there whenever dad was home. After mom passed away, I think Al spent most of his time there.

When it was mealtime, Al wanted to eat in his room but I insisted he and I were family and we needed to eat together. He did come out then. We ate pretty much in silence. He would then rinse his dishes, put them in the dishwasher and return to his room.

This felt so awkward to me. I was not used to eating alone when there was another person in the house. Eating like this continued for many months. I just had to get used to it. In fact, it got so stressful with no talking that I would eat in the living room and he ate at the kitchen table.

He seemed to like that better. He started speaking out more and we would talk from room to room. It was a long, long process but eventually we each adjusted to our strange way of sharing a meal.

On Friday nights, I went to my job. Either Al went to a ball game in town or he would go to an auction if there was one nearby. I felt a little uneasy knowing he was driving and I was at work. I had to trust that he would be alright. He had been forced independence years ago and I had to continue to let him do things on his own.

Saturday nights he went to an auction that was out-of-town. Because of his routine, the weather never came in his mind. He just knew it was Saturday and it was auction night. I used to worry while I was at work. I knew he was driving in the snow and I hoped he would be alright. Sunday mornings he went to church.

In my eyes, Al was never the perfect driver. He had a few accidents which thankfully what was damaged was non-living. It was the mentality that he and I challenged many times.

He drove the same speed always, slow. He took the same route no matter what the weather. He and I lived out in the country so there were many times the roads were bad. I would pray to get to my job safe and Al just knew his routine.

I am glad I let him do his thing when I look back. We don't know our future and sometimes as we sit and look back at what we have done, we can be thankful for some of our decisions.

Al and I were at home. I was in my bedroom and he in his. I was surprised when he entered my room. *I was thinking, wow this is great. He and I are going to spend some time together apart from meals.*

He smiled at me and continued to stand there. I started chatting with him and then suddenly he started shaking. I immediately stood up and asked him what was wrong. He didn't talk and the smile was gone.

I reached out to him and he partially collapsed in my arms. It turned out Al was having a seizure. I dealt with this and once I knew what was happening to him my training kicked in and I was able to keep him safe.

His seizure didn't last long and I helped him back to his room and helped him lay down on his bed. We made it through that night but first thing in the morning, I called his doctor. An appointment was set right away and I drove Al to the office. Al didn't even argue about me being the driver.

With some testing and conversation, Al had a big piece of information given to him and he was not happy about it. His driver's license was being revoked. Al could no longer drive.

I felt sick about it. Al had been independent for some time. This was not a choice. It was thrust upon him. Dad had a belief I didn't agree with. It was out of sight out of mind. Even when we were kids dad believed we should be seen but not heard.

So not being able to drive was another stab in his life. He had a rough life at times. He was the child that wasn't normal, but then again, what is normal? He had his heart attack. He was let go of his job and now his driving privileges had been taken away. I knew this was going to be a challenge to get through.

Chapter 20

The clouds hung lower and tension began to build in our home. I was busy trying to work with the attorney for the estate. Al was home all the time and seemed to spend a lot of time in his room.

I tried very hard to take him out every day. The seizure after-effects didn't last long. He was able to still do many things, but for Al, he thought his life was about over.

Our parents were gone. Our sister turned a corner and began to drift out of our lives. I had my three kids but something was missing. Joy is what I call it. For Al, it was a reason to continue on with each day.

Three families lived in separate houses on one property. An Aunt and Uncle had moved out of Indiana to Florida. Our wonderful Grandma had moved to Florida also. She was getting older and without my dad nearby, she needed more help than what any of us young ones could give her so she moved in with her daughter.

We began to hear more from our Aunt in Florida. Her family had moved there from Indiana when one of their children had Cystic Fibrosis. They had been relocated about 25 years it seemed like to me.

When our Grandma was still living up here Mary would come here and help begin the process of transferring her personal items and her to her home. I got the chance to talk and spend some time with her.

Once they were moved, our house seemed rather lonely. We drifted from one day to the next. I worked my weekends. Al ended up not being able to go to auctions on Saturdays since I was gone and he couldn't drive.

I started taking him to local auctions that were on Mondays. This seemed to help but I still felt sad for him. He had nothing to do on the weekends so stayed in his room more and more.

Our Aunt began calling. It soon became an everyday occurrence. She would call to check on Al and me and that felt good to know someone out there cared. Soon without even realizing it, the conversations turned to moving to Florida.

I couldn't think of that. My children were here, close to me. How could I move so many miles away from them? Nevertheless, as each day continued and people started drifting back to their normal lives from our dad's funeral, the thought of warm weather and a chance at a new life sounded interesting.

Mary and I began searching for properties. Something that was easy to maintain. Al couldn't mow and my Diabetic neuropathy stopped me from several things. She mentioned a condominium type living.

I chewed it over and I began to ask Al how he would feel about selling the homestead and making a fresh start. I was amazed at how eager he was to go. He told me," Living here has bad memories of Dad. I want to move out of here."

We discussed selling the home and moving into a different one in our own hometown, but it was winter and that brings snow and cold and the sound of warmth hit the spot. We both came to a decision, and that was to move.

I listed the house. It bothered me a great deal. Not so much the house itself. It didn't hold that many memories for me. I had never resided there and it was on five acres so I had to pay to have someone mow the property.

The house itself was very nice and the setting was beautiful, but still; it was missing something called family.

My daughter informed me not long that she and her husband would be moving out-of-state for a new job. I was devastated. She and I were so close. We hung out at each other's homes all the time. How was I going to survive without her? I couldn't wait for the house to sell.

I had the sadness of leaving life and memories behind. I had the thoughts of Al and how he felt about this home. I knew my daughter was leaving, and the biggest tug at my heart was; what would my dad say if he knew I was selling his home.

I had to keep in mind that dad was in heaven. I had to make choices according to how I was living at the present. So I just prayed daily. If we were making the right choice to move to Florida and not remain here, God would allow the house to sell.

God did do exactly this. The house was sold within one week. I was amazed. Look at how God had let this happen and so quick. I kept Al informed of everything that was going on. He and I spent more time looking at homes online and searching out things for him to do in the new city.

We looked at shorts and clothing suitable for warmer weather. Our time became consumed with moving. With the help of our Aunt, a condominium was located and we purchased it.

It was such a smooth transaction I just knew God had been the one in charge the entire time. Al and I began to make a list of things that needed to be done. So many things, such as boxes obtained, bank accounts transferred, and the estate was closed and finalized.

On a warm, sunny day, everything was loaded up and we said good-bye to our familiar territory.

Chapter 21

Al and I spent a night in a local hotel on our last night in Indiana. The next morning Al was very talkative and ready to get out-of-town. My daughter was here and she was driving us down. We ate breakfast, took one last look at the home property, and headed out on the highways.

Al was amazing. He did well on the trip. It was a 24-hour drive. He made me smile many times as I discovered he knew each license plate and what state they were from. There were times when he also knew the county the plate belonged to. This occupied him for the better part of the trip.

Al enjoyed stopping at restaurants and gas stations. Something new to look at and discover. We went past the huge Coca Cola plant in Georgia. Al was so excited to see that. I will always remember the Coca Cola plant.

I had contacted them one time and explained how Al was a big fan. The company sent him several souvenirs and invited him to take a tour. Although, we never got to do that, Al always treasured that package that came for him in the mail.

We arrived in Florida. It sure was hot. The truck arrived and they started unloading while we started trying to empty boxes. My daughter stayed for a few days but then went back to Indiana. I sure did miss her and after she left I cried like a big old baby.

It took quite a while to find our way around. The city we lived in was Sarasota and it was much bigger than our hometown. One good thing that came out of our scoping areas was I found a place Al could go to through the weekdays.

It was a place where disabled adults could hang out. They ate lunch there. They socialized and played pool. There were counselors that came in and spoke to each client.

The best thing that Al liked was getting to go on outings. Since the city was so big, many businesses donated tickets to different events. Al was fortunate to be able to go to several movies, plays and he ate out once a week and sometimes twice.

He got to go to Tampa to baseball games. He went to outlet malls in different towns and got to go shopping. He searched for Coca Cola in every flea market they visited. He sometimes went to Siesta Key beach and the group of them cleaned the beach of trash.

He was never crazy about doing that job but he went because he knew he would be with his friends. Al loved to talk. I always called him the social butterfly. Everyone knew Al and he seemed to never know a stranger.

The weeks turned into months and the sun seemed to be a big help to Al, but things never stay the same and one day he started having chest pains. I thought he was having another heart attack and so the EMS was called.

He wasn't having a heart attack but the doctors knew he was experiencing something real. They admitted him into the heart hospital. The doctors discovered he had new blockages but they were not bad enough for repair. They also learned he was experiencing heart angina.

He was released the next day and we just took it easy at home for a couple of days. There was nothing really to do for him, but I started keeping better mental notes of what was happening and how he acted.

More time went by. Al and I enjoyed some dinners with family and we learned of a great Amish restaurant. It was a buffet type and all the food was made from scratch. This place became Al and my favorite place to go.

Inside Dutch Heritage, they also had a section of reproduction and genuine antiques. Another part of the restaurant was a bakery. Al always made a stop in front of the glass and admired the sweet treats.

After a couple of visits, we found a little section that had day-old goodies and in no time, Al was picking out one thing to take home on every visit.

Oh, these memories make me smile. I had seen Al so sad and angry for so many years. It was a pure joy to my heart and soul to see him smile and talk and laugh. He had a full life. A life full of friendships, exciting places to go, and awesome places to eat.

One day Al had been to an evening outing. The bus brought him home and when he came in the door, he seemed fine but in a blink of an eye, everything changed. He looked at me as if he was seeing a ghost. He started to cry. He asked," Who are you? I don't know you and where am I"?

It scared the crap out of me. I had never seen him like this and I knew without a doubt he was playing no joke. I tried to tell him who I was and where we were but he was scared. I called the EMS and they came.

After numerous questions, they suspected Al had a seizure. They took him to the hospital and he was admitted once again. Several tests were done on him but each one came back negative.

A specialist for brain issues came to see Al. He wanted permission to do a special test. I was all for it as long as I knew Al was not going to suffer in the process. The doctor explained the procedure. Wires would be attached to Al's head and they would take a different type of picture that would go deeper inside the brain to see if they could find anything.

Chapter 22

The test was scheduled for the next day. Al asked a lot of questions but I assured him it was not going to hurt. I explained how they were just going to take a fancy picture of him. He seemed content with that.

I was there when the specialist arrived. He set everything up and explained the procedure to Al and me. After the wires were attached, he begins doing his magic. When it was all done, the doctor showed me what he had suspected.

Al had some brain damage happen from the seizure he had. He said that I should not be surprised if in the near future Al would begin to show Parkinson's disease as it was so strong in the family.

Al didn't seem to really understand and I explained as briefly as I could. I didn't want him to get this disease. I had seen the effects of it with three different family members. The specialist unhooked everything and left.

The next day Al was released and we went back to our normal routine of living. I tried to brush the doctor's words to the back of my mind. Why worry when he showed no signs of it.

About three months went by from that day at the hospital. I started noticing Al was tripping over himself. He fell a few times getting in and out of the truck. I tried telling him to be more careful, to walk slower, and not to be in such a hurry, but in the back of my mind, those stored words were starting to surface.

The next time he fell out of the truck was the last time. He not only cut his legs but he was limping. I called the family doctor and made an appointment to take him in. After seeing Al, he sent him to a sports doctor.

The new doctor did x-rays on Al's legs and he had torn ligaments in both knees. That was the last time Al rode in that truck. We went car shopping and got something that Al could get in and out of with ease.

Nothing stopped for him. The car made it easier but then a slight tremor started being seen in Al's one hand. It went from there to the upper arm and then on the same side the leg started to twitch.

Once again, I called the doctor. After checking him, he thought it best to send Al to a neurologist. He told me he was pretty sure Al had Parkinson's disease. I smiled at Al as the doctor spoke but inside I was screaming, no, no, no.

The appointment took a couple of weeks. In the mean time, Al didn't have the tremors too often. When he did have them, I could see they bothered Al. He always told me he was trying to get them to stop but he couldn't.

I started researching this nasty disease. Although I had been familiar with the word and had seen some of what it can do, I needed to know more. I didn't like what I read. I kept reading the same thing over and over, *no cure and gets gradually worse*. The worst I read was there was no cure and Al could suffer for years with this.

Upon arriving to the appointment, he had Al do different tests. Strength and walking, squeezing fingers, and gait. The doctor diagnosed the final words Parkinson's disease. He explained about exercise and how Al could benefit greatly from it. He explained how the tremors might spread from the one side to both sides. He said the head could shake or the lips tremor.

I shook his hand and thanked him for the insightful information. Everything was going to be different from now on. My family members had terrible tremors and one of them ended up in a wheel chair. I was going to make sure Al lived life and had as much fun as he could possibly have while he could.

There was nothing really prescribed for Al at that time. We made no special changes. We just waited and dealt with what he was given each day. The tremors did continue. They moved from the one side to both sides.

He didn't have the lip tremor and he didn't drool. Other than the shaking of the hands and legs, he led a pretty active life. I continued to allow him to go to his adult day care. I did not want him to have to think too much about the doctor's visits.

He was scheduled appointments every six months to see if the disease was progressing. Only then did we actually voice the word Parkinson. Al still went on the outings and seemed to be having a good time.

I then started hearing him complain about his hands. I had noticed they were shaking a little stronger than in the past. He was mad because he was beginning to lose control over them. He was beginning to spill things he was trying to hold.

I noticed that he would sit on his hands to get them to stop shaking. For some time that did seem to help. The more he seemed to struggle the more I began to spoil him. I took him out to eat all the time.

We went to the flea markets and shopping. Whatever clothes he wanted I tried to buy. We looked for coca cola items even harder. Life was still pretty good when I look back at it now.

He then began to complain of chest pains again. I took him back to the heart doctor and his exam showed him that Al was just stressed out from the shaking. He started prescribing calming medications. Before too long had passed, Al was on Parkinson's medications along with antidepressants and the calming medications.

Chapter 23

The calming medications helped a little with Al's issues of being frustrated with the tremors. The Parkinson's medications didn't help at all. Each visit I took Al back to the doctor, different PD medications would be tried, but none worked.

The doctor kept him on them though. I really wasn't happy with that. I have this thing about medications. If they don't work, get rid of them. We dealt with each day and I watched as his tremors progressed. Nothing else seemed to be happening in this illness.

Al continued to go to the adult day program and I tried to live as if nothing had changed. He went to this one outing where the clients all went to a discount mall. Afterwards they stopped to eat and when the bus driver brought him home, he stayed long enough to let me know that Al had seemed tired and had actually fallen asleep on the way home.

If you knew Al like I do you would know this wasn't something he would ever do. Al was such a social butterfly. He would fight sleepy eyes in order not to miss talking to one person.

I told the driver thank-you for the information. When I went inside to ask Al if he had a good time, he was already in bed with lights out. I wished him a good night's sleep and didn't mention what the driver had said.

The next morning seemed pretty normal. Al ate his breakfast but instead of watching the TV like he usually did on Saturday mornings, he wanted to lie down and nap. I thought this is odd. Al never misses the Three Stooges.

After he got up, he seemed back to normal. I asked him," Do you want to go to the flea market?" and he said yes. So we hopped in the car and drove the couple of miles. Al seemed happy. He smiled and talked to ever vendor. He found a couple of coca cola bottles and that seemed to make his day.

We didn't have any more issues for some time, but then things changed again. Al was having chest pains. I made another appointment at the heart doctor. After checking Al, he decided Al needed to be hospitalized to check for blockages.

Al wasn't crazy about this. He always commented," More needles?" He was getting used to being admitted I think. The test showed Al had more blood clots in his heart valves but the doctor said they were not big enough to remove. So along with this information and now knowing that he has Angina of the heart I was getting concerned for his health.

PD, heart issues, what was next? Al was a little more quiet when we arrived back home. He seemed a little more tired and slower in movement. When the following Monday arrived he wanted to go back to his Day Program, so I took him.

When I picked him up a staff member asked me to come in so we could talk. Al stayed in the rec room and I went into the office. The director said," We all love Al here at Day Program. He is such a nice guy; but we have rules. Everyone that attends here must know their medications and what they do for them. All must know their address and telephone number. We are not a babysitter service. We are here to oversee."

I had tried many times to get Al to repeat his address and phone number but he never got it. I couldn't understand why the Day Program felt it was important for the clients to know what medications he took and what they were for.

The Director explained", the clients that come here have:

Schizophrenia.

Schizophrenia (/ˌskɪtsəˈfrɛniə/ or /ˌskɪtsəˈfriːniə/) is a mental disorder often characterized by abnormal social behavior and failure to recognize what is real. Common symptoms include false beliefs, auditory hallucinations, confused or unclear thinking, inactivity, and reduced social engagement and emotional expression. Diagnosis is based on observed behavior and the person's reported experiences.

Clients with this diagnosis need to be aware of what they take and why so they can live a more productive life. Al does not have this diagnosis and we all voted for him to join us here since he is so nice. But now, he seems tired and he is starting to repeat himself. So we don't have time to keep a better eye on him, so we must ask you to not bring him back anymore."

I was devastated but I knew Al would be much more than that. Standing up to leave the director shook my hand, gave me his apologies, and said, "We sure will miss him."

I went in and found Al and said it was time to go home. I didn't mention the conversation all the way home. He went to his room and turned on the TV and I went about starting supper.

During supper, we were both quiet. Al didn't talk much unless I started the conversation when it was just us. He never could mentally separate me from our dad. Al and dad didn't get along at all. With dad not accepting Al for being someone other than the common word normal, there was much friction between the two all of Al's life.

Dad was short-tempered with Al. He wanted him to be quick to move and answer like most people. There were barely conversations between the two that were ever looked at as social.

Al looked at dad as the boss. When I started caring for my brother, I had to guide and teach him many times and Al looked at me as the boss. He could never separate the two people.

This was Al and my biggest issues in our living together. It hurt me so bad that Al couldn't see how much I loved him and wanted him to have fun and to be happy. Many, many times I would end up almost screaming at Al after a trying conversation that I was not dad, but me, Terry, his sister.

I would ask him," Do I look like dad?" He would begin to cry and say no. I would get frustrated and walk away. None of this changed until many months later.

Chapter 24

Life wasn't getting any easier. I decided Al needed to be home where his familiar doctors were. Al and I were not crazy about this idea. We both didn't really want to walk back into memories that upset Al and made me sad.

The house listed and before we realized it, we were packing up rooms, getting a moving van and were headed back to Indiana, our hometown. There was really no excitement between the two of us as we saw the Warsaw sign come into view.

It was late and we were both tired from the travel and all the things that go along with moving. Because of the friction that was heavy in the extended family, Al and I didn't let anyone know we were coming home except my kids.

My son was waiting on me to let me in to our new home. The movers were tired but went straight to work unloading the truck and setting up our beds. I believe Al and I finally flopped into bed around 4am.

The next day I wanted to pull my hair out as I looked around our home and saw box after box. Al and I both needed to take morning medications so we dug clothing out of our overnight bags, got dressed, and went into town for breakfast.

It didn't take long while eating that Al and I started talking about the past. Had people's views changed while we had been gone those few years? Was the talk about who was to get what past now that the estate had been closed long ago?

As we ate, we watched the news on the overhead TV and watched cars go by. Afterwards we went back to our home and Al started putting his room together. He complained of being tired and sore. I told him", Just do what you can bud. I will help you with everything else."

He seemed alright with that. He went for his prize coca-cola and started setting it around. Then he got his clothes out and put what he could in his drawers. He cleared off his bed and lay down to watch TV.

That was fine with me. He didn't feel well and yet he still helped. I spent most of the day busy putting things away. I started with the bathrooms and then the kitchen. I made sure that things we needed were unpacked first. Dishes, glasses, silverware, toilet paper, bath towels and wash cloths.

By the end of the day, I was exhausted but still not finished; but at least I had a path to walk through. Al and I ordered a pizza for supper and had it delivered. For the rest of the evening we watched TV and went to bed early.

The next day was more unpacking. Within three days, I had the place presentable. I then started on the projects for Al. I called his former doctors and had records sent here from Florida. I called a company that Al used to work through to see about a Day Program.

By the end of that day, we had scheduled appointments set with our new family doctor, Al's old heart doctor, and Cardinal Center, the company Al had been associated with for years.

We went to supper at Golden Coral. Al loved eating there because it was buffet and he could make all his own choices. Al did pretty good walking. His top half of his body leaned to the side and his total side definitely was weaker, but he got what he wanted to eat all by himself.

As the days moved forward, we discovered through the heart doctor that Al had suffered what is called a TIA, a silent stroke. This is what caused his upper half to lean to one side.

The heart doctor said for the damages that Al had suffered in his
heart attack and the Angina he had now, he was in pretty good
shape. She said he would not be able to keep us with most people
and he would tire more easily than others. I was happy with this
news.

The family doctor took Al's vitals and had his records from where
we had lived here before and his records from Florida. He asked
many questions such as how was Al feeling on a daily basis, how
was his appetite, did he suffer constipation, did he take vitamins.

After having an hour meeting, the doctor ordered a CBC, (complete
blood count) for Al and said to come back the following week.

We had only seen one neurologist when we had lived here prior but I
had actually forgotten that so a new doctor was ordered. We went to
see him a couple of weeks later.

We spent the in between hours enjoying the fall weather and looking
at pumpkin decorations and houses that were fixed up for
Halloween. We decorated our own home for the holidays and soon
drifted between doctor visits and the thoughts of Christmas and
snow. Neither of us was looking forward to that at all. I think this is
what we missed the most about Florida, no snow.

We ate out a few times a week. My son told Al and me of car shows
that were coming up. I decided to take Al to see them and before
long Al had decided to add a new interest to his hobbies; car
collecting.

My son loved Chevy Bel Airs. He had one that was aqua blue and
Al fell in love with it. Al started collecting these same types of cars.
If he could not find one, he would purchase an old car of another
model. He loved the police cars from the era of Andy Griffith. By

the end of Al's life, his room was filled up with these two special cars and many others along with his coca cola that he found.

Chapter 25

Our days were filled with trying to do things that Al loved, but Al's illness was doing something else. He began to fall. The first time he fell was in the hallway. There were tiled floors and the furnace was right there.

When he fell, he broke one of the tiles and knocked the front door of the furnace off. I was so scared he had injured himself but the only injury to him was fear. I helped him up and then with assistance we made it to the couch.

I offered him a coke after checking him all over. No blood and no lumps. While he was drinking his pop, I started talking to him about the fall. How he should begin to hang on to things as he walked.

I had our grandma's old cane here and offered it to him but with his stubborn pride, he refused it. We didn't experience any falls for about another month and then they became more frequent.

The big fall came near Christmas Time. He was walking to his bedroom and suddenly, with no warning he fell straight into the Christmas tree. This time I was scared. His head was turned sideways against the wall. I could see his legs but our tree was big so he was buried underneath all the leaves.

I told him," Don't be afraid bud, I am going to call 911 and have them help me get you out from under there. I am afraid I will hurt you if I try to move you alone." He seemed alright with that.

I called 911 and they came. Three EMT's recovered him from the branches. They took his vitals. His blood pressure was up a little but they thought that was from the accident. They talked to them, filled out paper work, and then left. I helped Al to lie down on his bed. I knew that he had enough for one day.

There was one other time that he had fallen. It was in his room and he was squeezed in between his bed and lift chair. I couldn't get him up and I saw blood on his forehead. I called 911 again and they responded immediately.

Al was alright. They placed a small bandage on his forehead and filled out another report. All of us put him in bed so he could rest. I walked the EMT's to the door and they stopped and told me something that scared the crap out of me.

They said that if they were called one more time they would have to by state law report this to the Adult Protective Services. I asked them why and they said," Your brother is mentally challenged, right?" I nodded yes." Anytime there are falls from someone like him, we have to report it on the third fall." I thanked them for their service and information and let them out.

Shutting the door after them, I walked to the couch, sat, and thought about how cool this was not. With the bad relationship between him and his dad, and now, both parents were deceased; I was all Al had left. I was his guardian and sister. I couldn't let anything happen that may take him away from me, but what could I do.

I mulled over this for days. Idea after idea came and went and then I knew that I needed more help with Al than what I could do myself. I also knew that I needed to protect him from being placed out of our home.

I began to call nursing homes. After finding one that seemed nice, I set an appointment for them to come meet Al. I dreaded so badly telling Al, but when I did at supper that night, he shocked me.

You have to remember his mentality. At that time, his intelligence was about 10 years old. He was very excited. He said," This is great. Look at all the new friends I will make and I can play Bingo."

I almost wept inside at his innocence but smiled. If he had to end up going, I wanted him to go with this attitude. No more falls happened within the next two days and when the doorbell rang early Monday morning, I answered it and let in the staff from the Nursing Home.

They wanted to meet Al and then after their little chat Al returned to his room to watch his favorite TV programs. Considering the time of day, he was probably going to watch the Price is Right show.

Many questions and answers is what I did for the next hour. By the time they stood up to, leave an appointment was set to bring Al into the nursing home for a tour. Al seemed very excited. I, on the other hand, was getting nervous. *Al not here with me? I don't know if I can deal with this. I am his sister and no one will ever love him, understand him and care for him as well as I could.* I kept thinking about how he could be taken out of this house and I had to do what I had to do to protect my brother.

The day came and we were getting ready to go in the front doors of the nursing home. Staff was there to show us around. I stayed in the background while they showered Al with attention and showed him the highlights of the place.

After the tour was over they asked Al," Do you want to come live here with us?" Al nodded yes. My heart broke but the fear inside me was bigger. I signed all the paper work and two days later Al was living in his semi-private room at a local nursing home.

Chapter 26

What I didn't expect to happen when Al moved into the nursing home was guilt. Guilt surrounded me. Everywhere I went, every thought I had; guilt was there eating me alive. I went to see Al almost every day for the six months he was in there.

I ate lunch with him each time. Sometimes I went for supper or breakfast. I had been in the nursing field for over twenty years so I made several non-routine visits. Everything seemed to go well the first few of weeks.

Lots of attention was showered on Al. Staff coming into his room more than I had had dreamed, but then things calmed down, and then the storms started to brew. When Al went into the nursing home, he could still walk with his cane.

Before Al had entered those big, front doors he had already spent three months here at home doing physical therapy with the staff from this nursing home. Al complained a lot from pain but I thought those old words, no pain, and no gain.

I requested that he have no more therapy once he entered the nursing home, but somehow my feelings were over looked and therapy became a constant in Al's life for the next several weeks.

What I didn't realize, but was beginning to recognize was the more Al did his workouts, the more tired he became. His bounce didn't come back like it does for the rest of us. With lots of studying and learning, I discovered that after a certain point of having MSA, the muscles do not bounce back. They have the reverse effect. They begin to crumble.

Of course, at this point I did not know that Al had MSA, (Multiple System Atrophy). I was under the assumption he had PD, Parkinson's disease. Al began to sleep more but I thought this was due to the illness.

What I learned though was staff quit paying attention to him. They came and helped him for sure, but the extra time was not there anymore. He was becoming bored. With his mentality at age 10, the older folks that reside in nursing homes just plain weren't keeping Al's interest.

He did enjoy Bingo. He won treats, which he kept stored up in his room. I always told him," You are storing these like squirrel stores nuts for the winter aren't you?" He would laugh and soon I discovered he was eating them at nights along with his bedtime treat staff gave him.

Now I always kept Al's dresser full of treats. Anything from Reese's cups, Twinkies, Granola bars, about anything he requested, and of course pop. It didn't take long to figure out what was going on when the staff began to let me know of Al's weight gains.

I had seen too many deaths in my career and always believed that if I was going to get a terminal illness, it was better to be on the heavier side. I know, this sounds crazy. We are supposed to eat lean and stay fit.

However, I saw things in a different light. Knowing Al had PD, I wanted him to be as happy and content as he possibly could. I should just come right out and say it, I spoiled him rotten.

I knew what PD could do to his life and so I was determined to make the rest of his days full of smiles. In the end, I was very thankful that Al had gained weight. It saved his life for a little extra time.

So, back to what I was talking about. When I noticed Al was getting weaker and learned the information I did, I demanded therapy quit working him so hard. They did listen to me and turned to an infrared machine that they would place on Al's sore muscles and help them to feel better.

They spent more time with him working his fingers to help them relax and stay flexible because of the nasty tremors. Al seemed to draw into himself a little more each day. I began to carry more guilt at how I was to blame for him being there, even if he did want to go.

I was about to go to the head of the company and make a request that I wanted to take him home for good. Before I could carry that thought out, staff came to me wanting to talk.

" I am afraid this is not working out. With Al's mentality and his attitude changing, I think he would be better off somewhere else." I agreed and thought how easy she had made my own speech for me.

What I didn't know is just in the changes he had already made it was going to be a little harder to care for him at home, than I thought. Thankfully, some caring staff members opened my eyes to waivers. I had never heard of these before.

After careful explanations about the several waivers there were, I decided on a particular one. The process began but it took three months, so Al had to remain there longer than I wished. The waiver I had chosen stipulated that the patient had to be in a nursing home in order to qualify for this certain waiver.

It was worth it though. When Al came home in June of last year, there were programs in place that allowed Al to be able to go out in the public with the aid of wheelchairs and ramps. When Al came home, he was tired. I could see how much weaker he had become since entering the nursing home. Part of it was due to being more restricted in a room than the outings and activities that he and I had shared here at home. The other part was the illness.

Chapter 27

It took a few days to get into a routine of caring for Al once again. With the help of some programs, we were able to get Al a lift chair. He loved it. He was able to get in and out of it without my assistance.

To me, no matter what illness you have, independence is something that should remain strong for as long as possible. The one company that had been in Al's life got involved with me and Al again.

With the help from the waiver, this company was able to provide a transit bus to come straight to our front door. Al could be taken out to the bus in his wheelchair and with the help of the lift on the bus; Al was able to go to the Day Program.

In the Day Program, Al could be social with others like himself. He ate the packed lunch I prepared with his friends. He made crafts and made plenty of friends. Soon this died down as Al became more tired.

When Al had still been in the nursing home, the staff recommended a Neurologist for Al to go see. This was for a second opinion. We went to the assigned appointment. Up until entering that door, I had totally forgotten that we had seen this doctor once before, years back after he had his heart attack.

When we were entered into the data system and shown which door to go into to wait to see the doctor, I was still a little leery of this doctor. After all, we had a Neurologist already. Our doctor was full of life, made Al feel at ease, and sometimes produced laughter from him.

On the other hand, I wasn't going to argue. Our Neurologist did not prescribe certain medications so Al was at a standstill. So maybe this doctor could add something to the recipe.

When the doctor walked in I recognized him immediately. How could my mind have slipped so badly? I place the blame on being a caregiver and dealing with so much all at the same time.

The doctor said hello and then turned to Al." How have you been since the last time I saw you Al? I can see there have been some significant changes since you were here before."

I didn't say anything to that remark. I guess I didn't want him to realize I had forgotten who he was. Al smiled but didn't say anything. By now, Al didn't talk near as much as he used to. It was quite alright for me to do his speaking for him, although he was right there beside me in the room.

After doing some tests on Al he looked at me and said, " I knew what was wrong with Al the first time he was here but I couldn't say what it was because there wasn't enough documentation per say. But now I am absolutely positive, your brother has MSA."

I shot a look at the doctor. I was so surprised to hear this. Oh not that he hadn't said these silent thoughts before but for the fact here I was in nursing for over 20 years. I had dealt with all types of illnesses in those years and had never heard of this.

I asked the doctor," What in the world is MSA?" He went on to explain," It is a neurological disease. It is similar to Parkinson's disease but there are a few major differences. For one, MSA, (Multiple System Atrophy) does not seem affected by the popular medications that are used for PD. Another difference is the brain loses contact with anything Al would want to do with his body. The memory stays intact with MSA. Rarely is it ever lost such as in a PD patient. The last thing is the life expectancy. PD patients can live many years with this disease, but for an MSA the average life span is six to seven years."

I looked at him but really didn't say much. I glanced at Al to see if he had caught much of what the doctor had said. I don't think he did. Al was more interested in going to lunch like I had promised him we would do after leaving here.

My mind was starting to roll like a train taking off on the tracks. What is he not telling me? What is this MSA for sure? I kept hearing six to seven years life expectancy. Looking back, Al had already had this terrible disease for five years now.

The doctor wrote some notes on a yellow sheet of paper and when Al and I were ready to leave the doctor handed me the paper. He patted me on the back and said," Read these notes. If there is anything or anyway I can be of help, please don't hesitate to let me know." I smiled and then wheeled Al to our car. We were off to lunch and I could tell from Al's actions and words the doctor's words didn't sink in.

We went to Al's favorite place, Zale's Pharmacy. Al and I had grown up there I should add. Our parents had gone there it seems forever, so everyone knew us. The staff always made Al feels so special. They waved at him each time he went in and said hello. Different people would sit and chat with him while we ate at the inside luncheonette.

This time though I didn't talk as much. I spent my free time reading the paper the doctor had given me. It pretty much said in easy words, that there was no cure for Al's disease. That this, disease could affect his already damaged heart. I was to make sure Al kept up with appointments at his heart doctor. The last thing he had written was how sorry he was that he had to give me this terrible news.

Chapter 28

This new diagnosis changed everything. Some ways that Al had been acting didn't seem right for what PD did. In a way, it was a relief to know that he now had MSA.

http://www.ninds.nih.gov/disorders/msa/detail_msa.htm

You can type this in your own search bar and get some information on MSA. I won't try to make you believe that you will find all the answers to your questions. There isn't a lot of information on this wicked disease.

From the day we got home from Zales, I began to be my own teacher. I studied for hours, days, and months. I read everything I could. I talked to people and doctors. It was disappointing to me that barely anyone in my own living area had ever heard of this.

I knew that the kind of person I was, I would dig in and come out knowing as much as anyone would allow me to soak in. I would be my brother's advocate, sister, and guardian. I thought I would always stay on top of this and be mentally and physically prepared for whatever was to come at us.

Of course, I was wrong. How can I actually know anymore than some doctors? Nevertheless, I did learn a lot. I belong to Face book and there are several member web pages that are full of people who have MSA.

Actually, I always felt honored to be included in the web pages. We became like family. I have several friends who are suffering from this disease or have family members who are. I felt and still do that most of those suffering from this terrible illness belong on Face book. You ask me why I think that. Because MSA, is so rare.

Multiple system atrophy has a prevalence of about 2 to 5 per 100,000 people.

People like Bonnie, and Carole, Janiece and Lise and Connie are among the dear friends I have made through Al's illness. I believe in the old saying, ***no matter what storm you are going through, there is a rainbow if you look hard enough to find it.***

This is the way I feel about these friends of mine. They are not just friends; they are a part of my life and family. With an illness this rare and this scary, you and I need all the support we can gather up. If you have MSA or know of someone who has it, please open an account on Face book and type in the words MSA. You will be happy with the information you find.

Want to know more about MSA? I will provide you with some information below.

The Multiple System Atrophy Coalition
8311 Brier Creek Parkway
Suite 105-434
Raleigh, NC 27617
vjames@msacoalition.org
http://www.multiple-system-atrophy.org 🖾
Tel: 1-866-737-5999

Who discovered MSA in the beginning?

http://pmj.bmj.com/content/77/908/379.full.pdf

Al and I fought through this wicked disease together. He continued to go to his Day Program from July 2013 through Halloween of 2013.

He had a Halloween party to attend to at the Day Program. He didn't want to wear a mask, which I didn't blame him or try to talk him into. Instead, he picked out his favorite coca-cola clothes, and this is what he wore.

When he was dropped off back here at home. The bus driver helped him down. She then asked me", Has anyone called you from his classroom?" I said no, and she suggested I get a hold of them.

There was still time before they closed so I got Al safely inside and placed him in his lift chair. By now, Al didn't walk anymore. After the strenuous therapy days, he just didn't have strength any longer. He didn't walk alone anymore. He went from the single cane, to a four-legged walker to now total help from me. He could stand long enough to pivot for me to get him in and out of his chair or in his bed.

I called the Day Program teacher and was fortunate enough to be able to speak to her before she headed home. She told me," Al cried throughout much of the day, and if he wasn't crying, he was sleeping."

Oh how my heart broke. Knowing that under any other circumstances, Al would have been the life of that party. To cry, because for Al, pain on some level was always present. We were never able to walk away from it.

Stronger medications were used for pain and all of Al's other medications were removed by the following week of the Halloween party. I knew things were very serious when the doctors decided to take away his heart medications.

I knew enough from my career training that the MSA was so strong within Al; the other medications he had taken to feel better and survive were no longer working. Now Al was only on a few medications. Very strong ones for pain in liquid patch and tablet forms.

Oh, how could I get through this? How could I remain strong and smiling for my brother when I knew his life was in jeopardy? By the strength of God, that's how I did it and he held on to my hand tight and guided me throughout the rest of Al's days.

Chapter 29

Each day Al got weaker, not only his body but also his mind. He was becoming confused. He complained a lot of not being able to see well. Twice in six months, I took him to see his eye doctor and I heard the same thing each time.

The muscles behind the eyes were not able to focus as well as before. This was causing poor vision. With Al's other medical problems there was nothing the doctor could do for him.

I could do something for him though and I did. I invested in a much bigger television for him. Every Sunday that I can remember, Al read his Bible, so I purchased him the largest print Bible I could find.

My heart just melted when I received the biggest smile from him. He could read it and he loved it. Al was a very routine oriented guy. I think most of this came from his mentality. He had grown up going to church and Sunday school on Sundays so when he could no longer go to church we both began to watch Joyce Meyers and Dr. Charles Stanley on the television.

Any other day of the week, he showed no interest in God. With the illness quickly progressing, I knew that it was time to try to change his view on routine. I explained to him that Joyce Meyers was on the TV six days per week. I told him", Bud, you even have choices. You can watch her in the mornings or in the evenings or both. Dr. Charles Stanley comes on twice on Sundays here. You can watch him in the morning and in the evening."

He seemed to like that idea and so each day I would turn his station to either him or her and gradually he also began to read his Bible daily. I really didn't have that much to do with this entire grand plan in his life. Al was able to read his Bible for a couple more months, and then I began to read to him since he could no longer focus. God helped life to become tolerable. I began to do something I had never thought of to do before.

I was determined that each day I would find something good about it. Whether it was seeing the sun peeking through a cloud or just watching the squirrels in our yard scrambling to find a piece of food, I would notice and I would smile.

By now, Hospice was involved. The waiver that had helped Al to come home provided help for me to care for Al. The illness was so strong that for a few months before Al passed away, I only went outside the house once a week and that was for groceries.

It is truly amazing when I look back to just a few months ago and see how much God had a hand in our lives. I had lost my father back in December of 2007. I began to care for Al in January of 2008, after his heart attack. I never began the mourning or healing process from our dad passing. I went straight to caring for Al.

It was a whirlwind of a life. It seemed that I had lost many friends from being inside so much and being out in the social world had vanished, but God sent angels to me and Al. Our caregivers were wonderful. Gina, Stacy, and Faye were so good to Al and they cared and listened to me and held my hand while I cried.

Hospice came twice a week up until the last few weeks. They seemed to care about Al so much. His favorite nurse that came, Al had known for so many years. Hospice had many patients to handle, so they were never here long enough for me, but hey, I wasn't the patient, but I felt like some days I was cracking up from his pain.

The Hospice always made sure Al had all the supplies that he needed. One thing about MSA is; it doesn't sit still. The stages move very quickly. I would just get used to doing things one way, and boom, I was having to learn something new or a new way of handling the situation.

Al suffered from catheter issues, almost being blind. He went from feeding himself, to using heavy-weighted silverware, to finger foods, to me having to feed him. Then we went to mechanical soft diets, then to foods that consisted of soup, ice cream, or puddings.

While the MSA was moving, forward and I could see so much on the outside, his insides were worsening also. He had big issues swallowing. He would try to swallow but the muscles in the throat were not working properly, so choking issues became huge. This is why the constant change of foods.

Being on such high doses of pain medications caused terrible issues with constipation. Every day he or I was asked if he went and more often than not, the Hospice nurse would have to help Al to clear the bowels.

Al's body became stiff through time. His limbs would not move with his help. Somehow, the tremors always were able to move though. I remember once for a short spell Al wanted to get out of his bed. He had been bedridden for about a month at this time.

He begged and begged. One day when the caregiver was there, she and I decided we had to show Al that he could no longer get up. She and I got on each side of him and sat him up on the edge of the bed.

Both of us were scared as we watched Al's body flop around like the commercial on TV where the fish is out of water. He had lost all control. Control of his urine, bowels, eating, just about everything he could ever do, he could not now.

She and I quickly laid him back down and got him covered up. I asked him," Do you still want to get out of bed?" He said softly, "no, never again".

Chapter 30

Now that I have told you where to go to find more information on MSA. I will tell you my personal experience with Al, my brother and what MSA did to both of our lives.

I was able to handle and I believe Al was too, most of the daily changes that happened along the way, until he became bedridden. The disease had already progressed quickly in my eyes but now we were not prepared for the fastest roller coaster in the world effect.

Being bedridden was something Al fought. He wanted to get up but we had shown him it was not possible. Hospice had brought him a regular hospital bed and after a few weeks of being in bed all, the time Al started getting sores.

He was changed in positions every two hours and sometimes every hour but his skin was breaking down anyways. All caregivers, including myself put lotion on him twice a day. We paid special attention to the elbows and heels of the feet. We used as many pillows as possible because if you use too many on an air mattress, the mattress can't do its job; but we were fighting a losing battle.

Hospice thought it was time to protect Al's skin so they suggested an air mattress. It was a little bit of a challenge though. Al could not sit up or help in any way to make the transition of mattresses, so the fire department was called.

We told them when the new mattress would be delivered and they arrived precisely at that time. With the help of four firemen and us caregivers, we were able to hoist Al into a Hoyer lift. We sat him in his lift chair and everyone went to work quickly to change mattresses.

Al was so weak his body curled up into a ball in his chair and he began to fall forward. A couple of us hung on to him to save him from injury and in no time, Al was transferred to his new mattress. I was so thankful for these people's help I couldn't say thank-you enough.

Al was not able to eat the foods that he needed to keep the skin healthy. By now, he was eating mashed potatoes, puddings, and ice cream. Al craved sherbet. It seemed I couldn't keep enough in the freezer. Sometimes volunteers from the community brought some over.

I think the cold foods felt good on Al's throat. When he swallowed, he reminded me of a turtle in the way his head and neck moved. I was concerned because although he was a mild diabetic, all these sweet treats may cause his sugars to rise sharply causing him more problems.

Hospice assured me this wouldn't happen since he wasn't getting that much food at this point. From that moment of relief to the end of his days, I gave him anything to eat that he could swallow.

His head had turned on its side and was locked in position. It was so tight in its place that it made it very difficult to shave him. His ear didn't get the air it needed so it became infected, with the disease eating a hole in his ear. We had Hospice medicating this daily, but it never left.

Al was not able to communicate any longer by talking. I do remember there were two times in the very last parts of his days that he by the grace of God spoke to me. He could sometimes still blink, although only half-blinks, it was a blink for yes or no answers.

He could no longer move any part of his body. He had a catheter at this point and after having this inserted for a few weeks it started to become infected. I think this is when everything started to go downhill fast.

The normal process of catheter care is to completely change the tubing and bag one time per month, with bag changes made more often, but I wanted the tubing changed more. You ask me why? The answer is with the naked eye we cannot see what is going on inside the body. We can only guess or assume.

One of the times the catheter was to be changed, the tubing would not come out. Each time it was attempted, Al would moan in pain. I cringed in fear and my heart melted for the brother I loved so much as I wondered how they were going to manage to retrieve it.

With as much patience as possible and gentle nudges, the tubing end on the inside of his penis did release, but it tore some tissue and the blood in the catheter bag appeared and never left for good. Hospice did its best but the MSA was boiling inside of Al.

I believe that Hospice felt if they were to change it more often, which is what I wanted, that there was a much higher risk of infection for him. I understood what they were saying but I stressed each day because I didn't want Al to have to go through any extra pain.

Al was on high doses of pain medications, which in turn caused constipation. It just never seemed to end in my eyes. I know it hurt him because when any of us would attempt to roll him to the opposite side, he would moan in pain when we placed our hands to close to the abdomen area.

Many times after I left his room, I wept. I prayed for Al's release of this terrible disease. When I thought nothing could get any worse, it did. Al could no longer eat the baby bites of sherbet. He could no longer use straws or anything I would try to get liquids inside his mouth.

I began to use syringes to give Al a drink. It had to be done very carefully and ever so slowly. He would choke if I gave it to him at any speed so slow was the way we went with everything for Al from that day forward.

Chapter 31

Al was not sleeping too much. He lost interest in the TV. He enjoyed hearing us read from the Bible to him. He no longer could listen to the earphones because of the damage to his ear.

His skin became sort of see-through color. His nail beds had been gray for many months but now his hands were turning grey. Nurses and I always checked his feet because sometimes as death appears the feet will change in color.

I would check Al over with a fine-tooth comb. I prayed for him to go to heaven but I fought for my own selfish reasons he would remain with me. I barely slept anymore. Except for the caregivers, I took care of Al myself for these past seven years. My own body was fighting in a survival mode. I was always and will remain ever so thankful for my best friend Lezlie, who came to stay with me. I am not sure how long she stayed but it was several weeks. This allowed me to vent, and cry and try to rest.

My heart squeezed so hard for I knew in my soul Al was leaving me. There were two times that I mentioned to you earlier that Al spoke to me. I have no doubt that God allowed this to happen because I needed to hear what he had to say.

The first time was when I was in the living room. I heard his voice and I about tripped over myself from shock that he had spoken and raced in there. He said," Do you see him?" I replied," No, I don't see anyone."

" Right there, right beside you, Jesus is here. He says it is time to go home and to tell you that I am going to be alright."

I grabbed his hand. *Oh, please hold on a second as I wipe my eyes. I can't see the words I am typing. It is so fresh in my mind and my heart is not yet healed. Alright, I am back.* I took his hand and held it and I spoke for the two of us to God. I thanked God for getting Al and me through this. I thanked him for keeping me strong.

Al was very concerned about his coca cola and car collection. He begged to die but he was fighting it not wanting to leave his possessions behind. I told him, you take with you whatever you want bud. God will make room." I think this made him feel better.

Pastors and Hospice staff, and I tried several times to help Al pass on to the other side, but he was afraid. He didn't know what to expect, but do any of us? Ideas had been exhausted. I believe that God planted an idea in my mind.

With Al's mentality, I went to his bedside. I told him I wanted to explain something to him. I started saying to him, "you know how you and I always took our vehicles into the garage to get their oil changed? Well this is what God wants you to do. Get a body change. He will heal you bud, and make everything new."

I saw tears flow down my brother's eyes. I knew I had said it in a way he understood. Al cried and I cried. I sat with Al for hours, just holding his hand. I had Christian music playing in the background, and when he seemed tired of that, I would put his favorite movie in the DVD player, A Christmas Story. Al would listen to that repeatedly.

He seemed to drift off so I left the room. I could barely walk from exhaustion, stress, and my aching heart. I had sat down for about a half-an-hour when I heard his voice the second time.

I walked in to his room and stood by his bed. I picked up his hand and gave it a kiss. He looked right at me and said," Sis, I know that you took good care of me. I appreciate it and I love you Sis. You should always remember that I love you."

I bawled like a big baby. All those seven years I was never sure if Al saw me, his sister, or his dad in me. We had struggled as I said in earlier chapters, so when he said this, it was the best gift I had ever received. I couldn't let go of his hand. I just kept stroking it. He drifted off to sleep once again.

I sat with him for a while and then went back to the living room. My friend was asleep in the bedroom and it was very late. I decided to rest on the couch. I dozed off and on. Every time I woke I went in and checked Al.

The skies lightened up and daybreak had broken. I got up and went into check on Al and he was gone. My brother was gone. I just broke into the biggest sobs I had ever experienced. I stood by his side whispering to him how much I loved him.

Today, it has been three months since my brother passed away. My heart still feels a huge void and my home is very quiet. Friends have appeared and are helping me to get back out into the world, but it is hard. Sometimes I can go out and do well. Other times I can't and I come home to cry in my pillow. By the grace of God and my family and friends, I shall get through this. I will never forget my dearest brother, and I will never forget what a cruel illness took his life. My purpose of writing this book is to help others to not be as afraid as I was.

Changes happen quickly. You cannot count sometimes from hour to hour what will happen. Make sure you tell your loved ones how much you care. Talk about the good things. Talk about the memories you shared together. Remember, the memory is not touched by MSA.

I love you Buddy. I miss you but I know you are saving a spot for me in heaven, just like you promised.